Praise for *Turbo Metabolism*

"With *Turbo Metabolism*, you can carry Pankaj Vij with you as a personal trainer, careful researcher, and model physician. A leader in culinary medicine and a doc who enthusiastically walks the talk, Dr. Vij prefers to help you change your lifestyle rather than have you simply lose weight temporarily. In this book, he helps you become a better, healthier, more energetic you."

— **John La Puma, MD,** founder of Chef Clinic and *New York Times*–bestselling author of *REFUEL*, *The RealAge Diet*, and *ChefMD's Big Book of Culinary Medicine*

"This wonderful work is the synthesis of the most effective, proven strategies for thriving. If you think no two experts agree, read this book. It will change your life."

— **Partha Nandi, MD, FACP,** author of *Ask Dr. Nandi: 5 Steps to Becoming Your Own #HealthHero for Longevity, Well-Being, and a Joyful Life*

"Dr. Vij has written an authoritative and exceptional book with great clarity. His wisdom and compassion come through in the effective strategies he offers to shepherd us toward a life of wellness, balance, and harmony. I highly recommend this gem of a book."

— **Sanjiv Chopra, MD, MACP,** author of *The Big Five* and professor of medicine, Harvard University

"*Turbo Metabolism* is the kind of book I'd like every one of my patients to read. By championing wellness through his superb understanding of metabolism, Dr. Vij gently but effectively coaches readers through the benefits of an anti-inflammatory diet, regular physical activity, and stress reduction. Readers will not only enhance their health but emerge joyful and feeling whole. I recommend it highly."

— Kavitha Chinnaiyan, MD, FACC, author of *The Heart of Wellness*

"Dr. Pankaj Vij unlocks the keys to metabolic health in *Turbo Metabolism*. His plant-based prescription has the power to save millions of lives and trillions of dollars in health-care spending, and to reinvigorate our medical system into a state in which wellness comes first."

— Neal Barnard, MD, FACC, author of
Dr. Neal Barnard's Program for Reversing Diabetes

"I am certain that *Turbo Metabolism* will be the catalyst to a movement toward healthier and more fulfilling lives. We are eating, sitting, and stressing ourselves to poor health and even early death, and we need to be slapped awake. *Turbo Metabolism* is the wake-up call to let you know that your grocer and personal trainer may be more important health allies than even your health-care provider. Read and implement the strategies in this book, and your health will bloom."

— Joel Kahn MD, FACC, author of *The Whole Heart Solution*

TURBO
METABOLISM

TURBO METABOLISM

8 Weeks to a New You:
Preventing and Reversing Diabetes, Obesity, Heart Disease,
and Other Metabolic Diseases by Treating the Causes

PANKAJ VIJ, MD, FACP

FOREWORD BY JOEL FUHRMAN, MD

New World Library
Novato, California

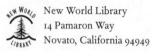

New World Library
14 Pamaron Way
Novato, California 94949

The material in this book is intended for education. It is not meant to take the place of diagnosis and treatment by a qualified medical practitioner or therapist. Please consult a qualified health-care practitioner before beginning any diet or exercise program. Any application of the material set forth in the following pages is at the reader's sole discretion and risk, and the author and publisher assume no responsibility for any actions taken either now or in the future. No expressed or implied guarantee of the effects of the use of the recommendations can be given or liability taken.

Text design by Tona Pearce Myers

Library of Congress Cataloging-in-Publication Data
Names: Vij, Pankaj K., [date]- author.
Title: Turbo metabolism : 8 weeks to a new you : preventing and reversing diabetes, obesity, heart disease, and other metabolic diseases by treating the causes / Pankaj K. Vij, MD, FACP ; foreword by Joel Fuhrman, MD.
Description: Novato, California : New World Library, [2018] | Includes bibliographical references and index.
Identifiers: LCCN 2017044312 (print) | LCCN 2017049843 (ebook) | ISBN 9781608684991 (Ebook) | ISBN 9781608684984 (alk. paper)
Subjects: LCSH: Metabolism—Disorders—Prevention—Popular works. | Metabolism—Disorders—Treatment—Popular works.
Classification: LCC RC627.54 (ebook) | LCC RC627.54 .V55 2018 (print) | DDC 616.3/90654—dc23
LC record available at https://lccn.loc.gov/2017044312

First printing, February 2018
ISBN 978-1-60868-498-4
Ebook ISBN 978-1-60868-499-1

Printed in Canada on 100% postconsumer-waste recycled paper

New World Library is proud to be a Gold Certified Environmentally Responsible Publisher. Publisher certification awarded by Green Press Initiative. www.greenpressinitiative.org

10   9   8   7   6   5   4   3   2   1

This is gratefully dedicated to all my patients who have had the courage to trust in the healing power of their own bodies.

Contents

Foreword

Now is the time to change your health destiny and finally get well. Remaining overweight and diabetic not only can kill you — it will also make you suffer needlessly for years. Modern nutritional science has shown that we can wipe out what I call these diseases of nutritional ignorance. Nutritional excellence can not only prevent cardiovascular illness but also reverse it, even in advanced cases. It can also reverse type 2 diabetes.

The finest doctors are master coaches who motivate their patients to adopt healthful practices that can enable self-healing. This describes Dr. Vij, an elite physician who stays up to date on the recent advances in science and is committed to your health and recovery. He is an example of a new breed of physician who addresses causation and avoids the needless and excessive use of medications and surgical procedures to treat chronic disease.

The underlying theme of this small but powerful book is that you can finally achieve a normal weight and keep the excess pounds off forever, no matter how many times you have failed in the past. If you follow Dr. Vij's guidance, you can achieve an astonishing health transformation.

We are fighting a war against obesity, diabetes, and chronic overeating. But the reality is that we have been losing that war to the food industry, which has hooked the masses on dangerous and addicting processed foods. The food industry promotes unhealthy foods and food-related behaviors to consumers, and it has billions of dollars to spend on supporting their aims. Sadly, they have been successful, to a large degree, in publicizing confusing, industry-promoted "science." This confusion leads to the failure of our population to adhere to a new paradigm of healthy eating. An overweight and sickly population serves the economic interests of the food and drug industry. However, in recent years, it has become more difficult to deny the overwhelming preponderance of evidence emanating from medical journals — evidence that is slowly enlisting a consensus among nutritional scientists.

People across America are misinformed and confused about health and nutrition. Until very recently, there has been mass confusion about what constitutes an ideal diet to prevent disease, normalize body weight, and maximally extend human life. Though there are outliers and deniers, who promote diets rich in oil or meat, most nutritional scientists are now in agreement that, for a diet to be considered health-promoting and physician-recommended, it must adhere to four basic tenets.

1. The diet must be rich in natural plant foods, particularly vegetables.
2. Carbohydrates should be naturally fiber-rich and low-glycemic, such as beans, squash, and steel-cut oats.
3. Salt, white flour, and sweeteners should be avoided.
4. Animal products should be significantly reduced.

Scientists throughout the world recognize today that low-nutrient calories, and excess calories, are toxic. When we overconsume calories, we shorten our lives and promote the development of chronic disease. In today's world, we have more people overconsuming calories to their detriment than we have people unable to find sufficient calories. It is clear that the shorter the waistline, the longer the lifeline — and the secret to a slim waist is more veggies and beans, not more meat and cheese.

One mass nutritional folly in the modern world is the idea of "healthy oils." Though there are healthy high-fat foods, such as sesame seeds and walnuts, there is no such thing as a healthy oil. For example, sesame oil and walnut oil do not have the cholesterol-lowering, heart-saving, and brain-saving effects that are associated with the whole nuts and seeds. Remember, oils do not grow on trees. They have never existed as a food for any animal on the face of the planet or for our prehistoric human ancestors, nor did they exist throughout most of human history. All oils are basically the same: They are heavily concentrated calories, with the natural fibers and most micronutrients removed. Oil consumption averages over four hundred calories a day for Americans and is a major contributor to our obesity epidemic. We need to eat less nutrient-poor calories and choose our calories and fats wisely.

Adding to this universal confusion is the idea that drugs are our answer to high blood pressure, diabetes, and high cholesterol, and that these medications will be needed for the rest of one's life. I feel strongly that if people knew the true risks of the medications they have been prescribed — and how little protection they offer — then millions more people would be embracing the nutrient-dense, plant-rich Nutritarian diet for the reversal of their health issues.

We have fantastic freedom in America, but that includes freedom to commit slow suicide with (fake) food. I think almost all nutritional scientists and nutritionally aware physicians agree that the American diet is a health disaster — one that has led to health-care costs that are completely out of control and unsustainable.

Our nation is suffering under the weight of a medical crisis that is difficult for most people to understand. While our government struggles to regulate health-care costs for a growing percentage of overweight, sickly, and medication-dependent people — and tries to find the most equitable way to do so — there is little conversation about the futility, the waste, and to put it simply, the damage caused by our nation's addictive dependency on drugs and medical care.

As a nation, we need less medical care, not more. We need to educate people about how to protect themselves from developing high blood pressure, diabetes, and heart disease. People need to understand that commercial baked goods, snack foods, and liquid soft drinks are as addictive and disease-causing as cocaine and cigarettes. Supervised abstinence is the key to freedom from dangerous addictions. It is important to recognize that cutting out sections of a person's stomach does not cure them if they are a sugar addict.

We have to come together and stop the insanity. We must say no to junk food. We must say no to processed foods and get back to gardening and eating closer to the Earth. We must fight for the survival and health of our fellow humans and make these changes together.

I hope you embrace this message and become an example for others to follow. Your health transformation will be a victory for all of us.

— Joel Fuhrman, MD, president of
the Nutritional Research Foundation and
New York Times–bestselling author of six books,
including *The End of Heart Disease*,
Eat to Live Cookbook, and *Super Immunity*

Why Turbo Metabolism, and What's in It for Me?

If you can dream it, you can achieve it.
— ZIG ZIGLAR

The two most important days in your life are the day you are born and the day you find out why.
— MARK TWAIN

Lights flashing and sirens blaring, the ambulance races toward the hospital. Inside the ambulance, Mary, a middle-aged woman, lies on a gurney, struggling with chest tightness, sweating, and dizziness.

Within an hour of her arrival at the hospital, Mary undergoes an angioplasty procedure: A wire is inserted into her occluded coronary artery, and then the artery is opened by inflating a small balloon inside. Finally, a "stent," which resembles the small spring inside a ballpoint pen, is inserted in the proximal, left anterior descending (LAD) artery (one of the heart's main arteries, a.k.a. the "widow-maker"), to prop it open permanently. Blood flow is restored to her heart. Several days later, she walks out of the hospital. The marvels of modern medicine have saved her life.

Though many catastrophic emergencies can now be treated with modern medical techniques, millions of people every year are still diagnosed with chronic diseases, such as diabetes, high blood pressure, heart disease, cancer, and stroke. And these diseases seem to be striking people at a younger and younger age. What is the cause of this epidemic? Do we simply need to have more ambulances and high-tech life-saving procedures? Or is there a deeper reason for this widespread problem? Why is it that the United States spends more money than any other nation on health care, yet it has the fattest, sickest population of any country in the world? Are we ignoring the root causes of chronic disease and simply trying to fix the problem by throwing money at it?

As I have pondered these questions, I have realized that many of my own relatives are in the same predicament as Mary. Even though most of them appear lean, with skinny faces, arms, and legs, they have visible belly fat — prominent bulges in their midsections — fitting the proverbial definition of "thin outside, fat inside" or TOFI, as it is commonly known.

At the same time, in my practice, I have observed that with just a little weight loss — as little as 7 percent of one's starting weight, or only ten, twenty, or thirty pounds for many people — my patients' need for blood pressure or diabetes medication can be drastically reduced. Even their heart-related symptoms can improve. As this occurs, they have a lot more fun and freedom. They can say yes to life's wonderful adventures more often and participate and engage in activities with their children and grandchildren.

I have often thought: Instead of treating a dangerous condition resulting from chronic disease, what if we implemented proven lifestyle changes before the disease reached the critical stage?

When I first started to scour the research, I found mentors in Dr. Joel Fuhrman and Dr. Neal Barnard, who were already working with thousands of people and helping them reverse chronic diseases and regain their vitality. Other really smart colleagues like Dr. Michael Roizen and Dr. Mladen Golubic were getting amazing results, while pushing for change at a policy level. I am immensely grateful to all of them for guiding the way and influencing my thinking about the reversibility of most chronic disease.

Thus, I started to experiment in using lifestyle optimization as the primary treatment for chronic disease. The results have been astounding. When we shift the focus to correcting the lifestyle factors that lead to disease, we are essentially treating the root cause. At that point, we can start thinking about prescription medications and procedures as a supplement to the first priority, which is treating the causes.

What are the five essential lifestyle ingredients that can reverse disease and add years and years to your life?

1. **Impeccable nutrition:** Eat enough highly nutritious foods that are not calorie dense. This maximizes nutritional content while minimizing empty calories. The food that we need provides fuel as well as information and intelligence from the environment, and it needs to be as nutritionally complete as possible. It needs to be satisfying and delicious because it is our most primal need. We need to be mindful of the toxins from the environment and to choose foods that minimize these toxins.

2. **Optimal hormone balance:** Eat the right foods and avoid hormonally dangerous ones (like dairy and alcohol). At the same time, make good lifestyle choices in terms of physical activity, stress management, meditation, and sleep habits to maintain optimal hormone balance.

3. **Regular exercise:** Move your body with joy and abandon as it is meant to be moved. Find enjoyable physical activities. Exercise also has benefits in terms of brain health — memory and mood — as well as heart health, metabolic, bone, and muscle health. Do you want to know the secret to Turbo Metabolism in three words? Activate big muscles.

4. **Stress management and quality sleep:** This combination is the foundation of a healthy lifestyle and the most critical emotional-resilience component of this book's strategy. Toxic load can also be caused by unmanaged repeated and prolonged psychosocial stress and lack of sleep. We need to be mindful of the importance of avoiding toxicity in our physical, psychological, and social environment as well.

5. **Social connections:** Loving, supportive relationships; meaning and purpose in life; and involvement in family and community can make a huge difference in health and longevity. Meaningful social connections help build *emotional resilience*, which is a foundation for healthy eating and active living.

When you start to master these five factors — of which nutritional excellence is the most important, lean muscle mass is the key, and emotional resilience is the foundation — you can improve your quality of life, reverse disease, and enhance your health.

Recipe for Disaster

Our typical diet might be the modern-day equivalent of a Trojan horse. It's as if an enemy wants to conquer us, and so they have encouraged our addiction to a diet of processed food loaded with sugar, fat, and salt and stripped of protective, natural disease-fighting superfoods (the "good stuff" found in plants that provides information and intelligence, not just calories). In this way, they are incapacitating a large proportion of our population with chronic disability and disease.

Currently, 70 percent of Americans are overweight or obese, and this number is projected to be even higher in the next decade, as childhood obesity, which has tripled in the last thirty years, continues to increase.[1] Over a hundred million Americans have diabetes or prediabetes, with increased risk of amputations, heart disease, and blindness.[2] This means almost half of our population either has "diabesity" (obesity with insulin resistance, prediabetes, or diabetes) or is getting there quickly.

This horrifying trend is also an urgent matter of economic viability and national security that should be part of the conversation on national policy right now. The United States has already lost its manufacturing base to China, and much of what we have left is the service industries. The 17 percent of our GDP (gross domestic product) that we spend on disease care is unsustainable.[3]

It is looking more and more probable that type 2 diabetes will become a global epidemic (with projections that one in three individuals worldwide will eventually be affected), as the rest of the world becomes more affluent, relinquishing their original diet of real food in favor of a more Westernized diet of processed junk mislabeled as food. Diabetes and metabolic diseases cost the United States over $245 billion a year, which exceeds the entire GDP of countries like Ireland, New Zealand, and Pakistan. Emerging economies like India now have 25 percent of the worldwide burden of metabolic diseases like diabetes and its accompanying curse of heart disease and strokes.

Right now, about 63 percent of US food intake is processed grains, and 25 percent is animal food, leaving a mere 12 percent for plant food — and half of this is processed plant food, like French fries, potato chips, and ketchup.[4]

Over 60 percent of our meals are prepared outside the home: When we let someone else take charge of our most vital interaction with the environment, we have no idea what we are being fed. Restaurant food is prepared to make it look and taste good, usually by adding lots of salt, sugar, and unhealthy fats.

Exacerbating the situation are the faulty US Department of Agriculture (USDA) one-size-fits-all, meat- and dairy-heavy nutrition models (such as the one listed at MyPlate.gov). These are less guides to a "balanced diet" than "broken plates." The USDA's primary job is to protect the interests of the agriculture industry, and these guidelines are fueled and funded by the dairy, beef, and grain lobbies. Certainly, this is well-intended advice, but the advice suffers from this inherent conflict of interest, and the unintended consequences have been disastrous.

The typical American eats "bit" foods — or "because it's there" foods — all day long. Donuts, candy, and processed "treats" are ubiquitous. However, the reality is that these are not treats; they are as dangerous and addictive as street drugs. The processed-food industry has figured out the formula for creating products that directly stimulate the reward centers of the brain (just like cocaine and heroin); as a result, the industry ensures that "You can't eat just *one*." Sadly, they are dead right, yet these substances are completely legal and socially acceptable.

Here's the bottom line: "Diabesity" (insulin resistance), prediabetes, type 2 diabetes, and obesity are human-made diseases. Some people may have been born with an increased genetic predisposition, but these conditions have manifested as a result of *personal decisions* — whether they were intentional or not. Genetics is like a loaded gun: It's up to you to pull the trigger. You are holding the solution literally in your own hands *right now*.

Insulin resistance and unleashed inflammation are at the core of most of the diseases of Western civilization. Having just a few extra pounds of weight, especially on your belly, starts this process.

Find Your Reasons Why

When you change your mind-set, you can develop the motivation and ability to change your destiny. Something triggered you to pick up this book. When you buy in to the idea with your heart and soul and set up your environment for success, nothing can hold you back from living the life of your dreams.

Are you going to let anything stand in the way of awakening your inner "superhero" and living the best life you can, starting right now? Self-examination is the first step.

What is the purpose of your life on Earth? Close your eyes for a moment and think about it. What kind of person would you like to be? What would you like to have? What would you like to offer to the world? What would you like to do, see, experience, and accomplish with your time and energy? What does your ideal universe look like in terms of your own self, your

relationships, and your finances? What does health have to do
with it? Why are you even reading this book?

If your goal is to live with meaning, purpose, and joy; to
spend time with loved ones and to make valuable contributions to the people in your community; to have more beautiful,
meaningful, and enjoyable experiences; and to learn new things
and grow and contribute, you will need to optimize your health
so that you have the vitality you need for this journey.

Autonomy, freedom to choose, and the pursuit of happiness are fundamental to our existence as independent beings,
and yet these basic rights can be snatched from us if we are not
healthy. So the goal of optimizing our "health span" is also fundamental to our existence. The end result should be more "life
in our years," that is, a longer health span.

What would *you* be willing to give for an additional five,
ten, or even fifteen years of vitality, productivity, fun, freedom,
and enjoyment?

We have a culture of short-term fads and cycles: January to
March is the time for making (and breaking!) New Year's res-
olutions. April to June is the period for crash diets, for getting
"ripped beach body abs and the perfect round tight booty" for
the upcoming summer. July to September is the time for summer picnics and vacations with pizza, beer, and chips. October
to December is the "holiday season" — watching football on
TV and eating lots of beef, pork, turkey, pie, cookies, and cake,
all washed down with alcoholic beverages wherever you go.

This book is not about the latest fad diet that might help
you lose twenty-one pounds in twenty-one days. It is about
changing your relationship with the environment. It's about
eliminating foods and habits that are making you weak and
tired and replacing them with foods and activities that make

you stronger. This includes optimizing food, water, and environmental exposures, as well as thought patterns. It's not about deprivation or sacrifice. Rather, it's about adopting an abundant new way of life that will give you the energy, vibrancy, and vitality that you deserve. It's about living life to the fullest, to enjoy every adventure life has to offer without any limitation or handicap, to be able to keep up with your kids and grandkids, and to say yes to more adventures, fun, and freedom!

Nutritional excellence, an active lifestyle, and emotional resilience form the three legs of the stool on which your health rests.

So, go ahead and be greedy! Create the perfect world for yourself, as you strive for optimal health: Taking care of yourself is the most profound way in which you can make a positive impact on the world around you. As the novelist Richard Bach states in *Illusions*, "You are never given a wish without also being given the power to make it true."[5]

How to Use This Book

This book follows my Turbo Metabolism program of diabetes and metabolic disease reversal, the same one I prescribe to my patients. The order of the chapters roughly corresponds to the way I present the material in my eight-week course, but it's not necessary to follow the program in the chapter order. Under the counsel of their personal physicians, readers can adapt the advice in this book to create their own health-promoting, disease-reversing program, one that fits their particular needs. However you use this guide, the final goal is to get rid of the things that make us fat, hungry, tired, and depressed and to awaken the "superhero" within!

For help defining for yourself why you want to make the commitment to better health, please turn to appendix 2, "Ten Reasons Why I Want to Achieve Turbo Metabolism."

RULES TO LIVE BY

- Fads won't change your life. Neither will pizza, hamburgers, hot dogs, and beer.
- Your purpose in life is far more important than your next trip to the refrigerator.
- Don't be satisfied with a recipe for disaster.
- Choose life. Invest in yourself.
- Nothing tastes as good as lean feels.
- There is nothing selfish about self-care.

Your Amazing Body

Your body is an amazing creation with an amazing ability to heal itself:

- Nerve impulses to and from the brain travel as fast as 170 miles per hour.
- The human body is estimated to have sixty thousand miles of blood vessels.
- Scientists have counted over five hundred different liver functions.
- Your nose can remember fifty thousand different scents.
- You use two hundred muscles to take one step.

- Approximately fifty trillion cells make up the human body.
- Every day an adult body produces three hundred billion new cells, completely renewing itself every seven years.
- The surface area of your gut can equal the size of a tennis court.

CHAPTER ONE

Metabolic Syndrome: The Root Cause of Chronic Disease

I wish I had a better metabolism. But someone else probably wishes they could walk into a room and make friends with everyone like I can. You always want what someone else has.

— KELLY CLARKSON

Let's start with some basic terminology.

Metabolism is a broad term that refers to the sum total of an organism's energy-producing and energy-utilizing reactions.

Glucose is the primary fuel in the body that is utilized by your brain, heart, kidneys, muscles, liver, and all the vital organs. The goal is to have lots of energy by having the *right* amount of the *right* kind of fuel available at the *right* time. Glucose is the *only* fuel that red blood cells can use and is the preferred brain fuel under most conditions. Muscles are the largest glucose-burning tissue in the body. The amazing thing is that the entire bloodstream can only hold three to four teaspoons of glucose at a time. This means that blood-glucose levels need to be tightly regulated at all times.

Insulin acts as the fuel injector that pushes glucose to the vital tissues for use as fuel. The problem with insulin is that when it is too high for too long, it makes us voraciously hungry and shuts down fat burning.

All carbohydrates eventually break down into glucose, which is the simplest form of fuel. *Sucrose* is table sugar, *fructose* is fruit sugar, *lactose* is milk sugar, and the list goes on. You are hardwired to seek out sugar because it provides energy. The goal is to find ways to provide this energy from *healthy* fuel sources, the way nature intended. In nature, sugar comes pre-packaged with fiber and water to provide a steady flow of fuel to the cells in the body. We interfere with this system at our peril.

Metabolic imbalances and diseases arise when there is a problem with fuel availability and utilization. This condition can be analogized to your car engine being flooded and then sputtering and producing soot and smog because fuel cannot be properly delivered and converted into energy.

So, metabolic disease is an energy-delivery problem at its core. To use another analogy, it's like having plenty of money in the bank but still being broke because your accounts are "frozen" or you are locked out for not having the right password.

Turbo Metabolism

Turbo Metabolism means having a properly functioning energy-delivery system, so that fuel is delivered and utilized optimally, providing plenty of energy for fueling a vibrant life. The result is a long and energetic life free of the chronic diseases that plague modern urban society.

The underlying cause of much metabolic disease is *metabolic syndrome* — the name for a group of risk factors that triples your risk for heart disease, increases fivefold your risk for diabetes, and causes many other health problems, including stroke, liver damage, cancers, sleep apnea, high blood pressure, and even chronic pain.[1] (*Risk factors* are traits, conditions, or habits that increase your chances of developing a disease.)

In obesity, the storage capacity of fat (adipose) tissue can be exceeded. When this happens, the excess fat accumulates in other tissues, which can cause them to malfunction. When the pancreas, muscles, liver, and cells lining the blood vessels are saturated with fat, metabolic syndrome may result (see figure 1.1).[2]

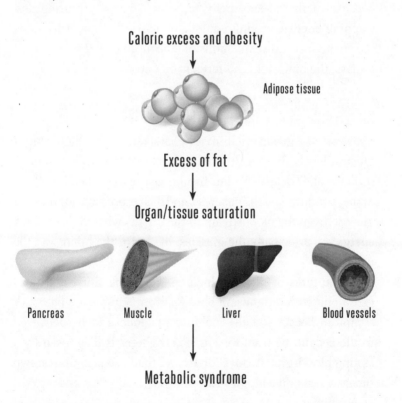

Figure 1.1. The process by which caloric excess and obesity lead to belly fat and metabolic syndrome

A telltale sign of metabolic syndrome is belly fat: the ugly fat cells that engulf our vital organs and surround the loops of our intestines. This is not the fat under the skin that can be sucked out during liposuction. It is internal, and the only way to get rid of it is by adopting the Turbo Metabolism lifestyle. Belly fat is very evident in people with a "beer belly" and is the source of all metabolic diseases.

The proliferation of this "hungry fat" makes us crave even more of the wrong foods. Think about it: You don't become overweight because you are hungry; you actually feel hungry because of this greedy belly fat, which keeps capturing and trapping energy, leaving you even hungrier! Thus, belly fat is the enemy of Turbo Metabolism: The more belly fat you accumulate, the hungrier (and fatter) you get!

Type 1 and Type 2 Diabetes

Diabetes is a group of diseases characterized by high blood-glucose levels that result from defects in the body's ability to produce and/or use insulin. Insulin is a master chemical (hormone) produced by the pancreas, and it is responsible for moving glucose from the bloodstream to the organs where it is used for energy — principally the muscles, the heart, the brain, and the liver.

Symptoms of diabetes include increasing thirst and hunger, along with fatigue and blurry vision. Fatigue is a hallmark symptom because of the inability of glucose to be delivered to the cells to be used for energy. Diabetes is diagnosed by a fasting blood-glucose level of greater than 126 mg/dL (on two separate tests) or a blood-glucose level greater than 200 mg/dL at any time.

Type 1 diabetes, which accounts for only 10 percent of diabetes cases, is caused by a deficiency of insulin production by the beta cells of the pancreas. That is, type 1 diabetics lack insulin, and they tend to be very thin and have a hard time gaining weight. *Type 2 diabetes* accounts for 90 percent of all diabetes cases. It is caused by *insulin resistance* — the body produces sufficient insulin, but the insulin is unable to work properly. The result is higher-than-normal levels of blood glucose because the glucose is unable to be processed by the cells and used for energy, so it remains in the bloodstream. When we measure insulin levels in type 2 diabetics, we find their insulin levels are actually very high, meaning that the body is compensating for insulin resistance by producing even more insulin! One of the big problems with chronically elevated insulin levels is that they cause constant hunger, and fat cannot be used as a fuel as long as insulin levels are elevated. As a result, type 2 diabetics tend to be heavy. The goal of Turbo Metabolism is to improve insulin sensitivity so that these soaring insulin levels can drop down to normal.

Heart disease, cancer, lung disease, stroke, and diabetes are the leading killers of our time and account for two-thirds of all deaths. According to the Centers for Disease Control (CDC), the percentages of total deaths by the seven leading causes are as follows:

1. Heart disease: 24.1 percent
2. Cancer: 22.7 percent
3. Chronic lower-respiratory diseases: 5.9 percent
4. Accidents (unintentional injuries): 5.6 percent
5. Stroke (cerebrovascular diseases): 5.3 percent
6. Alzheimer's disease: 4.9 percent
7. Diabetes: 3.0 percent[3]

If you are a nonsmoker over the age of forty, you can further narrow down the causes of death and disability to heart disease, strokes, cancer, and Alzheimer's disease. These are all characterized by impaired metabolism (problematic energy delivery) at their core.

If you really think about it, the actual causes of death underlying these diseases can be boiled down to a handful of largely preventable lifestyle choices, such as tobacco use, poor diet, and physical inactivity, all translating to impaired energy transactions in the body (impaired metabolism). Many of these lifestyle choices or behaviors stem from unmanaged stress, lack of social support, and poor sleeping habits.

In fact, the manifestation of a disease such as diabetes is simply the tip of the iceberg. Many decades before disease becomes evident, sinister "conspiracies" are brewing. Insulin receptors are becoming blocked and inflammatory chemicals are poisoning our vital organs and metabolic processes as a result of our behavior and choices. Essentially, we are gradually overwhelming the balance of nature. Using our car analogy, we are "gunking up" the engine, slowly plugging our intricately designed valves and fuel injectors, through the choices we make with our forks, fingers, and feet. The channels of glucose transport — that is, fuel delivery to the cells — are quite literally blocked by fat! Eventually, we completely overwhelm the body's capacity to cleanse itself; the scales are tipped and we are diagnosed with a disease.

The root cause underlying the problem is the excess of calorie-dense, nutrient-poor, toxic stuff masquerading as food, which essentially blocks the insulin receptors on the muscles and the liver and in the blood vessels. This causes serious difficulty with fuel delivery and utilization, incapacitating our energy-delivery system. These tissues essentially become "accessory fuel tanks" as we live in a constant state of feast without giving the system a chance to burn off the extra fuel.

Table 1.1 summarizes how physicians diagnose metabolic syndrome. Increased waist circumference plus any two of the criteria in the table results in the diagnosis. Metabolic syndrome is so dangerous because abdominal obesity (midsection or "belly" fat) produces harmful substances that cause inflammation and damage circulation and internal organs.

As stated above, your entire bloodstream can only handle three to four teaspoons of sugar at a time. Actually, the total amount of sugar you should consume in a day is zero teaspoons because refined sugar does not exist in nature. The body can extract all the sugar it needs from real unprocessed plant foods.

Table 1.1. Diagnosis of metabolic syndrome (a diagnosis includes increased waist circumference and any two other risk factors)

Risk factor	Measurement
Increased waist circumference	Greater than 35 inches (female), or 40 inches (male)
Fasting blood glucose	Greater than 99 mg/dL
Blood pressure	Greater than 130/85
Low HDL (good) cholesterol	Less than 50 mg/dL (female), less than 40 mg/dL (male)
High triglycerides	Greater than 150

The Role of Insulin

Insulin is the glucose-disposal hormone that is designed to move sugar from your bloodstream to your muscles to be used as energy. In fact, muscle is the largest insulin-sensitive tissue in the body. So one way to increase insulin sensitivity is to activate your muscles! Using our car analogy, insulin acts as the fuel injectors, supplying glucose (fuel) to the engine (muscles, brain, and other vital organs). Our insulin level soars when we both consume a high-calorie, low-nutrient diet — a diet high in manufactured, processed food that is mostly refined carbohydrates (sugar, high-fructose corn syrup, and white flour) and unhealthy fat (feedlot meat, cheese, industrially prepared vegetable oils) and low in fiber and micronutrients — and couple it with a sedentary lifestyle, high stress, and lack of sleep. In response to constantly elevated insulin levels, the cells, tissues, and organs become *insulin resistant* or insensitive. This is like how we "tune out" and no longer hear a constant sound, like a fan or traffic outside our window.

As shown in figure 1.2, constant and repeated spiking of blood glucose from a toxic diet of highly processed foods loaded with refined carbohydrates (such as from refined grain flours, sugar, and high-fructose corn syrup) leads to a constant elevation of insulin levels. With repeated glucose spikes, insulin levels have no chance to retreat to normal levels. This constant elevation of insulin makes us constantly hungry and leads to metabolic syndrome and type 2 diabetes. Thus, the formula is, repeated glucose spikes cause constant elevation in insulin levels, which leads to constant hunger and eventually disease. The key is to eat foods that release glucose slowly so that insulin levels stay low.

To summarize, in the presence of high levels of insulin, fat cannot be broken down into free fatty acids to be used for energy. This means that as long as you continue to consume a diet high in sugar and processed carbohydrates, your body will not be able to go to "fat-burning" mode. Thus, persistent elevation of insulin causes high levels of circulating blood glucose as well as fat accumulation. It also starts a perpetual cycle of hunger and cravings for sugar and high-glycemic foods (processed grains = fast carbohydrates = sugar releasing). The glycemic index is the degree to which food is processed to glucose in the body (for a chart of specific foods, see appendix 4). To hop off this cycle, your goal should be to follow a lifestyle that calms these raging insulin levels. Low insulin levels translate to less hunger, fewer weight problems, more fat burn, and less illness. When we provide the body with the right fuel, we begin to correct the hormone imbalances that wreak havoc on the entire system.

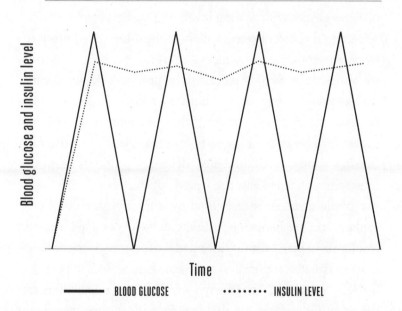

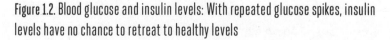

Figure 1.2. Blood glucose and insulin levels: With repeated glucose spikes, insulin levels have no chance to retreat to healthy levels

Insulin Resistance

You may wonder: How exactly does it happen that belly fat causes insulin resistance? Here's how.

In a series of unfortunate events, our modern diet — typically high in sugar, refined starches, and "dirty fat," such as trans fats and industrially produced oils — plugs the fuel injectors so that glucose can no longer enter the cells. Instead, glucose levels start to mount in the bloodstream. Muscle cells become insulin resistant, initially allowing energy to be stored as fat around the vital organs and in and around the liver. Eventually, these tissues also become insulin resistant. Thus starts the vicious cycle in which belly fat produces insulin resistance, and insulin resistance causes even more belly fat. As the liver and fat tissues also become insulin resistant, full-blown type 2 diabetes ensues with soaring levels of blood glucose.

Central obesity (excess weight in the midsection) produces hormones and other substances that are huge contributors to insulin resistance. Simply put, belly fat produces substances that act like a wad of bubble gum blocking a keyhole. Even though we have the right key (insulin), the door remains locked, and sugar is unable to enter the cells. It remains in the bloodstream, causing damage. Additionally, belly fat produces hormone messengers that make us tired, achy, and sick.

While diabetes is diagnosed by a fasting glucose of over 126 mg/dL, prediabetes is fasting glucose over 99 mg/dL, and insulin resistance starts at fasting glucose above 85 mg/dL.

Prediabetes and insulin resistance can precede type 2 diabetes by a decade. This is why I say that type 2 diabetes is just the tip of the iceberg. By the time we notice it, the main body of the iceberg has existed below our awareness for years. The result can be organ damage, such as eye and nerve damage, and its accompanying complications of full-blown heart disease and kidney disease.

Sugar Glazing, or the Importance of HbA1c

When we experience insulin resistance and too much blood sugar remains in the bloodstream, it causes "sugar glazing" of the hemoglobin in red blood cells. This is called *glycation*, and it results in glycosylated hemoglobin (also known as glycohemoglobin) or HbA1c. That is, a high level of circulating blood sugar makes the cells in the body, and the vessels through which they flow, "sticky." Imagine blood cells as Ping-Pong balls flowing through a pipe. Now imagine that the balls and the pipes have been dipped in honey. As they try to flow through the pipes, they damage the lining.

This glycation or "sugar glazing" causes cellular dysfunction and tissue inflammation, leading to degenerative diseases from oxidative stress. In fact, type 2 diabetes is the perfect model for rapid aging.

Advanced glycation end products (aptly abbreviated as AGEs) make not only the red blood cells but all the proteins in the body sticky. They are like the sticky fingers of a toddler, affecting everything they touch. When proteins are sticky, they can no longer properly communicate with one another, leading to the onset of dysfunctions that we typically attribute to aging. In fact, this process of producing advanced glycation end products causes proteins to malfunction and accelerates the aging process.

Indeed, did you know that Alzheimer's dementia is increasingly believed to be another manifestation of insulin resistance, one that affects the brain instead of other organs? Some investigators have even described it as "type 3 diabetes."[4] It should come as no surprise that the same metabolic conditions that cause heart attacks, strokes, erectile dysfunction, kidney failure, and amputations may also be poisonous to the brain! On the flip side, the lifestyle changes of Turbo Metabolism are also good for your brain.

The HbA1c Blood Test

In the HbA1c blood test, red blood cells are used because they can be extracted when we draw blood, and they have a life span of 90 to 120 days. Thus, the amount of sugar glazing or stickiness on them will depend on the blood sugar level for the last three months or so. Table 1.2 shows the correspondence between the HbA1c blood test and average blood glucose levels over the past ninety days.

Table 1.2. HbA1c test and blood glucose

HbA1c	Blood glucose (mg/dL)
5%	90
6%	120
7%	150
8%	180
9%	210
10%	240
11%	270

We know from research that a 1 percent reduction in HbA1c corresponds to about a 20 percent reduction in the risk of heart attacks and strokes and close to a 40 percent reduction in the risk of kidney, nerve, and eye damage.[5] Though most diabetes medications reduce HbA1c by about 1 percent, they do nothing for the underlying cause, so the disease progresses over time. When we start to understand the cause of diabetes, and act upon what we know, we not only *stop* the disease's progression, we can reverse most of its harmful effects, improving the HbA1c blood test by a lot more than prescription drugs. Table 1.3 shows some HbA1c levels and corresponding glucose levels.

Table 1.3. HbA1c percentage and diabetes

	HbA1c %	Fasting glucose (mg/dL)	Post-meal glucose (mg/dL)
Diabetes	>6.5	>126	>200
Prediabetes	5.7–6.4	100–125	140–199
Normal	About 5	<99	<139

CASE STUDY: JOHN

John, a sixty-six-year-old retired firefighter, was diagnosed as a type 2 diabetic with an HbA1c score of 9.5 percent. He was prescribed medications, but he avoided taking them. He had an aversion to testing procedures. Then, John joined the Turbo Metabolism program, and getting this information empowered him to take charge of his health. Now, John fully understands how his decisions directly affect his body, and he is much more mindful of what he eats. He also exercises regularly. His most recent HbA1c was 6.9 percent, and he feels much better. He recently returned from a hike to Machu Picchu in Peru, which is something he could not have imagined even a year before.

The Effects of Cortisol

Another hormone critical in insulin resistance is *cortisol*. Cortisol is a "stress hormone" secreted by the adrenal glands in response to a perceived threat. An integral part of our fight-or-flight stress response, cortisol provides a necessary bump in available blood glucose so that we have the energy needed to react quickly in an emergency.

Cortisol makes us hungrier, especially for calorie-dense, sugary, and fatty foods, and it increases insulin resistance, thereby increasing glucose levels in the bloodstream. It also contributes to belly fat. Cortisol is an example of a short-term survival mechanism kicking in to keep us alive in high-stress situations, but one that has harmful effects if it remains active — that is, if our cortisol levels remain elevated for a prolonged period of time in response to perceived stress.

The combination of high levels of cortisol and high levels of insulin is ideal for creating midsection or belly fat. Chapter 7 discusses the effect of stress as a contributor to metabolic diseases in more detail.

Inflammation

Another important concept is *inflammation*, which may be defined as the process of increased blood flow to an injured body part to deliver healing nutrients and infection-fighting white blood cells. Inflammation is characterized by swelling, heat, redness, and pain, and it typically occurs when we twist an ankle or stub our toe.

Many scientists and doctors accept chronic inflammation as the basis of most of our chronic disease and even of the aging process. The reality, however, is that short-term inflammation serves an important purpose in keeping us healthy. Have you ever bit your cheek eating dinner and woken up amazed the next morning because the cut has healed overnight? This is the miraculous, innate healing power of our bodies — our inflammatory response sends a SWAT team of infection-fighting white blood cells that secrete infection-fighting chemical signals to heal the wound.

This healing process goes haywire when we bombard the body with unrecognizable substances in the form of a diet rich in processed foods, sugar, fat, salt, high-fructose corn syrup, and synthetic compounds. The body activates the inflammation response, essentially sensing a five-alarm fire, and it continues this every day, so the inflammation response goes on and on. In other words, the body sends a SWAT team on an endless mission, so that it never leaves!

By the way, stress works the same way. An acute stressor followed by a short-term inflammation response is natural. But chronic, unmanaged stress leading to long-term inflammation can be harmful. For more on this, see chapter 7.

Hormone Imbalances from Excess Belly Fat

As I've said, insulin resistance, cortisol, inflammation, and belly fat are a direct result of our modern, unhealthy diet. In addition, lack of regular physical activity, chronic stress, and lack of sleep are also major contributors.

Yet there is another serious issue with belly fat: It is an active hormone-signaling system that wreaks havoc on our appetite, our cravings, and even our endocrine system — the network of hormone signals that allows our body organs to act in harmony.

In men, belly fat contains *aromatase*, an enzyme that converts testosterone to estrogen, which is bad news for men because men need testosterone for energy, vitality, maintaining healthy metabolism, erections, and libido.[6]

In women, excess belly fat signals the ovaries to produce more testosterone, which contributes to acne, hair loss, cysts on the ovaries, and lack of ovulation (also known as polycystic ovary syndrome, to use fancy doctor words). This is an important factor behind infertility and menstrual irregularity in women. It is in fact very common for supposedly infertile women to be able to conceive after losing some of their excess weight.[7]

Yet another problem with a diet loaded with processed foods full of carbohydrates and fats is that it triggers resistance to *leptin*, a satiety hormone. This resistance to leptin helps create the perception that we are starving, even as we are being overloaded with calorie-dense fake foods.

The Difference between Real Hunger and Craving

Your goal should be to maintain satiety or satisfaction, to start thinking about food as a source of energy and wisdom from nature. However, to understand satiety, you must first understand hunger. What does hunger mean to you? Craving sugar, chocolate, cheese, or meat is less likely real hunger and more likely an addiction reaction, arising from the effect of these substances on the reward center of the brain. The same sensations of craving — jitteriness, headaches, fatigue, irritability — are present in drug withdrawal. True hunger is a mouth or throat sensation similar to thirst. We often mistake thirst, boredom, nutritional deficiency, or a low blood sugar for hunger.

Have you ever been truly hungry?

A good gauge of whether a meal is truly nourishing is the degree to which it keeps you satiated. A meal that is biochemically suited to your needs should keep you satisfied for three to five hours.

In the following chapters, we will come up with a "zero-belly strategy" to turbocharge your metabolism, by exploiting the healing power that each of us is blessed with the day we are born.

Shedding ugly belly fat can be the key to reversing diabetes, improving heart health and memory, increasing energy and vitality, improving erectile dysfunction, preventing cancer, and getting rid of sleep apnea and fatty liver disease, in addition to injecting you with more energy and zest for life.

When your body is given the right fuel, you gain energy and vitality, and there is no need for it to be hoarded as fat in places where it can cause harm.

Every time you eat or drink, you are either nourishing your body or feeding disease. You have two choices: You can either "try" — that is, make excuses and then fail — or you can succeed no matter what obstacles come your way.

In the words of Yoda in *Star Wars*: "Do or do not.... There is no try."

Facts and Fallacies

- Fat is just inert excess energy.

  I I I I ■■■➡ Fallacy

  We know now that fat is actually metabolically and normally active tissue that produces insulin resistance, inflammation, and cravings for unhealthy foods.

- You cannot grow new fat cells as an adult.

  I I I I ■■■➡ Fallacy

  The reality is that you can grow new fat cells (and new muscle cells and brain cells) as an adult. New cell formation is called hyperplasia. *Enlargement of existing cells is called* hypertrophy.

- Being hungry all the time makes you fat.

  I I I I ■■■➡ Fallacy

  It's almost the reverse: Carrying unhealthy belly fat makes you hungry. Belly fat hoards energy (rather than releasing it for burning), leaving you feeling hungry all the time.

CASE STUDY: MARY

Mary, a fifty-three-year-old schoolteacher, had a long history of excessive weight gain. She had tried several weight-loss programs with little success. Entering the Turbo Metabolism program was a game changer for her. She began to think about food as energy and information. I emphasized that physical activity and emotional well-being were also very important, and so she incorporated strategies for both aspects in her daily routines.

In the process Mary dropped twelve pounds and three inches of fat from her waist in two months. She feels that these results are just the beginning, and she continues to feel better every day. By taking better care of herself, Mary has already had a positive impact on her students and colleagues.

RULES TO LIVE BY

Time for a reality check: Do you have extra pounds around your belly? Has your doctor advised you to lose weight, but you avoid tests, ignore test results, or prefer to pretend that you are not at risk?

Embrace a zero-belly strategy with these rules to live by:

- The battle is won or lost hand to mouth. What and how much you eat matters.
- Food is not the enemy. Substances *disguised as* food are the land mines to avoid.
- You can win this war. Once you recognize the problem, you can begin the fight against metabolic syndrome.
- The stakes are high. The food you put in your mouth today will determine the quality of the rest of your life.

CHAPTER TWO

A Holistic Approach toward the Treatment and Cure for Diabesity

This life's five windows of the soul
Distort the Heavens from pole to pole
And leads you to believe a lie
When we see with, *not through, the eye.*

— WILLIAM BLAKE

We are spiritual beings living in human physical form. Although most of us identify with our physical body, our capacity to thrive depends on so much more. The physical body is an amazing arrangement of natural elements, but it is virtually worthless without the vital life force that makes the body's roughly fifty trillion cells work together to form dynamic, creative, energetic beings, capable of doing so much good.

Vedanta philosophy (*veda* means "knowledge") describes this vital life force as *prana*, which stays constant even as we progress through different phases of life.[1] The Rig Veda is believed by historians to be the oldest available document in human history, dated from 10,000 to 4000 BCE. Prana, the vital

33

life force, connects the physical body to the mind — to our discerning intellect, knowledge, and wisdom, which help us distinguish the right path from the often-easier wrong one. Prana helps us to consciously make the right choices every moment of every day so that we can reach or remain in a state of balance and bliss with the universe, when we live life in perfect harmony and congruence with our own values and with nature.

Our foolish misidentification with the physical body is the root cause of overindulgence in sense gratification, through excessive consumption of food, drink, smoking, and drugs. This foolishness also leads to overattachment, which translates to destructive emotions, such as lust, anger, greed, arrogance, and possessiveness.

When we look beyond the physical body and realize that there is so much more to us than our five physical senses, we can connect with the ever-powerful, all-knowing forces of nature that are continually helping us heal and find balance and bliss. We can then realize that there is actually no "space" between us and the vital forces of nature. We, and everything around us, are made up of the five elements of fire, water, earth, air, and ether (or space).

If diabesity is a state of energy imbalance due to overconsumption, Turbo Metabolism is a state of harmony between the mind, body, and universe. This state of harmony can only be achieved by understanding and optimizing the free flow of energy throughout all three.

In ancient Indian philosophical texts, prana or life force is described as energy that should flow freely throughout the body through psychic centers of energy, documented as chakras as early as 800 BCE.

The Sanskrit word *chakra* literally translates as "wheel" or "disk." In yoga, meditation, and Ayurveda, this term refers to wheels of energy (or life force) throughout the body. There are seven main chakras, which are roughly lined up along the spine, starting from the base of the spine through to the crown of the head.[2] They are roughly aligned with the spine but can be visualized in the front of the body as well. To visualize a chakra in the body, imagine a swirling wheel of energy where matter and consciousness meet. This invisible energy, called prana, is the vital life force that keeps us vibrant, healthy, and alive.

According to WebMD, Ayurvedic medicine — also known as Ayurveda — is one of the world's oldest holistic (whole-body) healing systems. It was developed thousands of years ago in India.

Based on the belief that health and wellness depend on a delicate balance between the mind, body, and spirit, the primary focus of Ayurvedic medicine is to promote good health, rather than fight disease. But treatments may be recommended for specific health problems and are unique to each individual based on their mind-body constitution.

Yoga and Ayurveda are essentially inseparable sisters. Although yoga makes most people think of poses where people twist themselves like pretzels, its fundamental tenets are an eightfold system of universal morality, personal observances, postures, breath control, mastery over the senses, concentration, devotion, and ultimately, union with the divine. Hence, yoga is much more of a way of living than merely a practice of poses.

The Chakras: Energy Flow in the Body

The chakras, these swirling wheels of energy, correspond to massive nerve centers in the body. Each of the seven main chakras contains bundles of nerves and major organs as well as our psychological, emotional, and spiritual states of being. This life energy is always moving: We are living in a dynamic system that is constantly in motion, rebalancing itself, repairing, and healing all the time. Thus, it is essential that our seven main chakras stay open, aligned, and fluid. If there is a blockage, energy cannot flow. Another way to think about this is in terms of our personal growth and evolution. As we mature from infancy to adolescence to young adulthood, and from adulthood onward to middle age and beyond, we become wiser and priorities change. Our worldview changes, as do our needs. Growth and healing happens wherever energy flows. Energy flow requires awareness.

Awareness neutralizes some of the rigidity of fixed ways of thinking and keeps energy flowing smoothly. It allows us to understand when to hold on to things and when to let go. It creates the ability to choose consciously rather than acting in automatic, predictable ways. Because mind, body, soul, and spirit are intimately connected, awareness of an imbalance in one area will help bring the others back into balance. This shift in our mental paradigm is what is required for us to adopt a new way of living.

The Three Chakras of Matter

The first three chakras, starting at the base of the spine, are chakras of matter. They are more physical in nature. These chakras can also be thought of as symbolic of our most basic needs for survival — food, water, and shelter — and body organ functions, such as the capacity to excrete waste and to reproduce. These are dominant in our infancy and childhood, as the top priority at that time is to survive.

First chakra: The chakra of survival, stability, security, and our basic needs, the first chakra encompasses the base of the spine, the bladder, and the colon. When this chakra is open, we feel safe and fearless. It is the energy of feeling connected to the Earth in a way that is safe and nurturing. Having issues with safety and security can lead to problems with addiction to foods or money, or hoarding behavior that attempts to compensate for lack of safety and security at some prior point in life.

Second chakra: The second chakra is our sensuality, creativity, and sexual center. It is located above the pubic bone, below the navel, and is responsible for our creative expression. Issues related to sensuality and creative expression at any stage in life can lead to imbalances in our sexuality, such as insecurities, dysfunctions, or sex addictions later in life.

Third chakra: The third chakra is located in the area from the navel to the breast bone: the pit of the stomach. The third chakra is our source of personal power, our self-worth and determination. This is the seat of the "fire in the belly" that drives us to move forward. Imbalances at this level can lead to overidentification with the ego, manifesting as arrogance. This energy may be most powerful during our adolescent and teenage years.

The Four Chakras of Spirit

These chakras speak to our higher needs of truth, freedom, enlightenment, and bliss.

Fourth chakra: Located at the heart center, at the middle of the seven chakras, the fourth chakra unites the lower chakras of matter with the upper chakras of spirit. The fourth is spiritual in nature but serves as a bridge between our body, mind, emotions, and spirit. The heart chakra is our source of love and connection. It is at the level of the heart that we can expand the body horizontally. Think of it as opening your arms to hug or hold hands with a loved one or to hold hands with the people on your sides.

When we work through our first three physical chakras and into the fourth chakra of love and connection, we can open the spiritual chakras more completely. Our need for connection manifests itself in young adulthood as the most powerful. As we move and mature through adulthood, getting wiser, our needs change, as should our awareness.

Fifth chakra: The fifth chakra, located in the area of the throat, is our source of communication, verbal expression, and the ability to speak our highest truth. The fifth chakra includes the neck, thyroid, and parathyroid glands, jaw, mouth, and tongue.

Sixth chakra: The sixth chakra is located between the eyebrows. It is also referred to as the "third eye" chakra. It is our center of intuition. We all have a sense of intuition, though we may not listen to it or heed its warnings. Focusing on opening the sixth chakra will help you hone this ability, thus making choices that are in alignment with your values.

Seventh chakra: The seventh chakra, or the "thousand-petal lotus chakra," is located at the crown of the head. This is the chakra of enlightenment and spiritual connection to our higher selves, others, and ultimately, the universal divine.

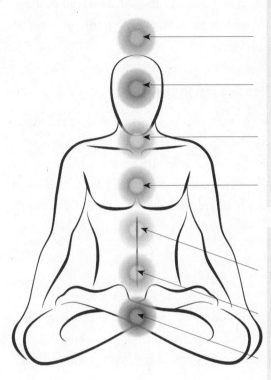

CHAKRAS OF SPIRIT

SEVENTH CHAKRA
Spirituality

SIXTH CHAKRA
Intuition

FIFTH CHAKRA
Communication

FOURTH CHAKRA
Love and connection

CHAKRAS OF MATTER

THIRD CHAKRA
Power

SECOND CHAKRA
Sexuality

FIRST CHAKRA
Survival

Figure 2.1. The seven chakras

Awareness: A Powerful Tool for Aligning the Chakras

Being aware when your chakras are out of balance is the key to aligning them. Our bodies are in constant flux between balance and imbalance. Unless you have an apparent problem in one area of the body, imbalances can be difficult to detect. That being said, building awareness of your body-mind connection is a good start in learning its signals and clues.[3] Awareness is a way to find equanimity in the midst of the perturbations of life. By becoming aware of where we might be stuck in our thinking, by adopting a mindful attitude and a relaxed posture, we can allow energy to flow more freely. Yoga and meditation show the way to achieve this.

Maslow's Hierarchy of Needs

When we are focused only on our physical needs, energy is unable to flow freely to help us achieve balance between physical and emotional/spiritual needs. Of course, this does not mean that physical needs are unimportant. In fact, as posited by Abraham Maslow, human beings have a hierarchy of needs composed of five levels, from basic survival needs to self-actualization:

1. **Survival**: food, shelter, and clothing (base chakra)
2. **Safety**: both physical and economic (base chakra)
3. **Love and belonging**: friendship, intimacy (middle chakra)
4. **Esteem**: confidence and achievement (higher chakra)
5. **Self-actualization**: achieving one's full purpose with creativity (highest chakra)

Physical needs related to survival and safety need to be met first before moving up to love, belonging, esteem, and self-actualization. When we feel threatened, we revert back to our survival and safety needs. When this happens, our focus is on hoarding energy to survive: Appetite is increased, especially for calorie-dense foods loaded with sugar and fat, and the body enters the mode of being thrifty so that the energy "burn rate" is slowed down. Thus, the impairment of metabolism that leads to diabesity results from the state of feeling threatened and shifting into overeating, energy hoarding, and "thrifty metabolism survival mode."

The ancient yoga philosophy — which first systematically

documented the chakra system in 800 BCE — long ago figured out what Western philosophers found out in the early twentieth century. The chakras correlate closely with Maslow's hierarchy of needs. The base chakras are concerned with survival and sexuality, which is the base of the pyramid in Maslow's hierarchy! The love and communication chakras around the middle (heart and throat) correlate with the love, belonging, and esteem portion of Maslow's hierarchy. The crown and brow chakras of spirituality and intuition correlate with "self-actualization," which was described by Maslow as the highest need.

Of course, these days, we might relate to an even deeper, more basic need than all the others: the need for Wi-Fi. I've modified Maslow's pyramid accordingly!

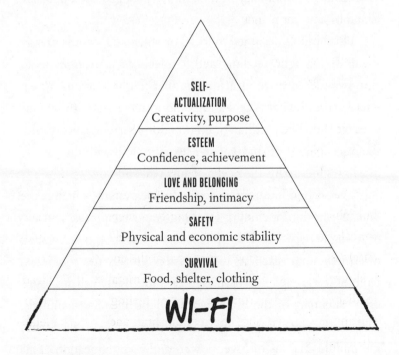

Figure 2.2. Maslow's Hierarchy of Needs

The Triune Brain Model

According to the triune model of the human brain, first theorized by American neuroscientist Paul MacLean in the 1960s and described in his 1990 book *The Triune Brain in Evolution*, we actually have not one but three brains, or at least three independently functioning parts of the brain active at all times. We need to understand and master all of them to achieve Turbo Metabolism.

The most primitive part of the brain, the hypothalamus and brain stem, controls things like appetite, temperature regulation, and the survival instincts. This reptilian brain is designed to help us stay alive, and we could not live without it. Our "survival brain" would kick in if we were dropped on a desolate island or another planet.

This brain is designed to focus on the four F-words of survival: flight, fight, feeding, and fornication. It prompts us to run away from or to fight threats that might harm us, to eat whatever and whenever we can, and to have sex with whomever we can. The reptilian brain functions correlate nicely with the base chakras of survival and sexuality and with the base of Maslow's hierarchy, the needs of survival and safety.

The second brain refers to the limbic system, which is the seat of emotion, including fear, rage, and happiness, and everything in between. This system also relates to our automatic, often irrational reactions and decisions: to eat the cookies in front of us, to engage in road rage, to impulsively yell at a loved one. This part of the brain can be found in most mammals, such as cats, dogs, horses, and chimpanzees. This correlates with the middle chakras of love, power, and communication. This would correlate with the emotional needs for belonging, love, and esteem in Maslow's hierarchy.

The most recently developed part of the brain, the neocortex, is the site for abstract reasoning, processing, and long-term memory. The cortex makes up one-third of the human brain and is unique to more evolved species, such as some species of dolphins. In humans, this part of the brain does not fully develop until the age of twenty-five and is needed for making decisions that involve delayed gratification, things that may feel difficult in the short-term but beneficial in the long-term. This correlates with the highest chakras of intuition and spirituality. When we operate at the level of the neocortex, we make thoughtful, pragmatic decisions that take into account all the ramifications of our actions. Mind mastery is all about operating at this level, or having willful control of the decision-making system all the time.

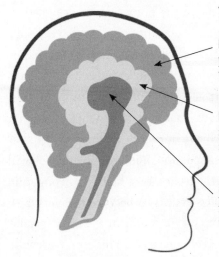

THREE BRAINS IN ONE

NEOCORTEX: Thought (including planning, language, logic and will, awareness)

LIMBIC SYSTEM: Emotion (feelings, relationships, nurturing, images and dreams, play)

REPTILIAN BRAIN: Instinct (survival, breathing/swallowing/heartbeat, startle response)

Figure 2.3. The triune brain

Rewiring Your Hardware and Software

With awareness, we can reset our hardware and operating system so that we can acquire the beliefs and the skills needed to achieve our goals. To paraphrase master coach Tony Robbins, Turbo Metabolism is about story, state, and strategy. To achieve Turbo Metabolism, you must first and foremost believe in and tell yourself the right story: the belief in self-efficacy (the idea that you actually have control over your destiny) and in your own personal effectiveness. When the right story gets paired with the right mental state, we position ourselves to do great things. After that, it is simply a matter of finding the best strategy, our most effective techniques, and nothing is impossible.

You shift toward a healthier relationship with food and the world around you. The strategies and skills needed for achieving Turbo Metabolism are learning to shop for, plan, prepare, and cook the right foods that nourish us with the energy and intelligence of nature; to move the body as it is designed to move; to get enough rest and relaxation; and to have a supportive social environment — all while steering clear of toxins. These beliefs and skills obviously require our complete emotional buy-in and a supportive environment (for more on this, see chapter 3). Our software, that is, our systems for living, the attitudes required to achieve our highest potential — positive thinking, optimism, compassion, and benevolence — will help us become self-reliant, autonomous, healthy, strong, and vibrant agents for good. The goal is to become the very best versions of ourselves.

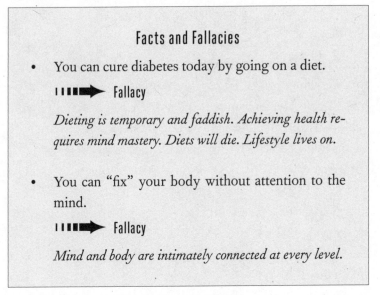

Facts and Fallacies

- You can cure diabetes today by going on a diet.

  ⊪⇒ Fallacy

  Dieting is temporary and faddish. Achieving health requires mind mastery. Diets will die. Lifestyle lives on.

- You can "fix" your body without attention to the mind.

  ⊪⇒ Fallacy

  Mind and body are intimately connected at every level.

RULES TO LIVE BY

- Develop awareness to uncover mind traps.
- Connect with the Earth to reestablish firm grounding in safety and security.
- Mind your thoughts because your whole body is eavesdropping. Your thoughts determine your destiny.
- Heal old wounds with attention, positivity, and optimism.
- Stop making excuses about past experiences and move on.
- Maslow's hierarchy and the triune model of the brain confirm what the ancient wisdom of the chakra system tells us: our personal evolution requires awareness so that we can achieve self-realization, which is our highest need.

CHAPTER THREE

The Nuts and Bolts of Getting Started

If you do what you've always done, you'll get what you've always gotten.
— TONY ROBBINS

To love oneself is the beginning of a lifelong romance.
— OSCAR WILDE

If you are still reading this book, the rest of my job is going to be easy. Once the "why" becomes clear, explaining what to do is straightforward.

One of the best urological surgeons in the country once told me, "I don't do anything special, I just cut and stitch all day — the magic of healing is in the body itself."

In fact, it takes a lot of effort to overwhelm the healing system of the body. Still, we've found the perfect recipe for disaster in our modern disease-promoting lifestyle of caloric excess, which originated with toxic substances mislabeled as food and has been coupled with unmanaged stress and a lack of physical activity and sleep.

When you put the *right* fuel in your body, health and

healing happen almost automatically. You are "designed" to move naturally. You do not need to do anything drastic. My program simply asks you to eat, move, and live in the unique way that you are designed to do. Everything else will take care of itself because the wisdom of healing is within.

The reason you need to get started right now is that the sooner you follow the right path, the easier it will be to heal. The further you go the wrong way, the greater the effort required to correct course.

Eating for health — rather than eating for entertainment — should be a conscious commitment.

Taking responsibility and affirming our control and autonomy, which is what we do when we consciously decide to nurture and nourish ourselves, are as applicable here as in other aspects of our life.

When we have been addicted to an unhealthy lifestyle, it takes time and effort to break the addiction. In fact, it can take up to forty-five days to take an idea from cognition (understanding) to emotional buy-in and finally to actual behavior change.[1]

The goal is to live in sync with our natural rhythms in an effortless way. This can happen as we move to convert our surroundings and routine so that healthy habits become our default. Think about a child learning to tie his or her shoelaces: The process goes from not knowing how to do it, to learning the steps, to practicing the steps, to finally being able to do it reflexively, without even thinking about it.

And here is the good news: The rewards — of more energy, vitality, and zest for life — are almost immediate. Although a complete transformation takes months, within a week or two, the taste buds start to adjust and the body starts to respond in such a way that you will not want to regress to previous unhealthy habits. The compliments you will get from friends, family, and coworkers will be a bonus.

Establishing Test Baselines

As you begin your journey to turbocharge your metabolism, it is important to track your metabolic numbers from the beginning so that you have a basis for comparison on later tests.

The first tests to start with are a fasting lipid panel — which includes total cholesterol, triglycerides, HDL (healthy) cholesterol, and LDL (bad) cholesterol — plus fasting blood glucose and HbA1c. The goal is to get total cholesterol around 150 mg/dL, triglycerides as close to 75 mg/dL as possible, HDL above 50 mg/dL, and LDL below 100 mg/dL (see table 3.1). Your fasting blood-glucose goal is to get under 75 mg/dL, and the HbA1c goal is under 5 percent (an ideal HbA1c is 4.8 percent). These tests are available and typically covered by most health-care insurance programs.

Table 3.1. Basic fasting lipid panel test with optimum levels

Test	Ideal levels
Total cholesterol	Around 150 mg/dL
Triglycerides	75 mg/dL
HDL	As high as possible above 50 mg/dL
LDL	Below 100 mg/dL
Fasting glucose	Below 75 mg/dL
HbA1c	Below 5%

Remember, these numbers are indirect markers of how well you have hit the state of Turbo Metabolism, where your body has all the energy it needs to do everything you ask it to do! As a Turbo Metabolism champion, you will most likely enjoy life to the fullest with all the great experiences, learning opportunities, and adventures that you deserve to have!

Supplementary tests may also be important in achieving Turbo Metabolism, depending on your specific health situation: high-sensitivity CRP (or cardio CRP), liver enzyme (ALT), thyroid-stimulating hormone (TSH), and vitamin D. See table 3.2 for the ideal ranges for each, and consult with your physician about adding these baseline tests.

Table 3.2. Supplementary baseline tests

Test	Ideal levels
High-sensitivity CRP (cardio CRP)	Under 1 mg/L
Liver enzyme (ALT)	Under 30 U/L
Thyroid-stimulating hormone (TSH)	0.1 to 3.0 micro IU/mL
Vitamin D	40 to 60 ng/mL

Preparing for Your Journey

Here are some tips to help you launch your journey to Turbo Metabolism. These actions prepare you mentally to succeed:

- Make a list of your personal goals by filling out the sheet "Ten Reasons Why I Want to Achieve Turbo Metabolism" in appendix 2.
- Announce your plan to several friends and family members, which will help create personal and social accountability.
- Ask a friend or partner specifically to support and encourage you. Even better: Ask the person to embark on this journey with you.
- Take nude photographs of yourself, front and side pose. Use these for a visual comparison as you make progress toward your goal (but keep them in a secure place and away from social media like Facebook, Twitter, and Instagram!).
- If you are diabetic, commit to testing your blood sugar levels after fasting, before meals, and sixty minutes after each meal. This is the only way you can gauge your own unique response to different foods.
- Make a list of nonfood-related activities that bring you pleasure, such as music, movies, comedy, being outdoors, getting a massage, or getting a manicure or pedicure.

Next, here are the first five action steps to take. The first three are described more fully in the rest of this chapter:

1. Take out the trash.
2. Shop for health.
3. Hack your bad habits.
4. Start a daily food log, listing the foods you eat each day.
5. Start an exercise log, listing your physical activities each day (see chapter 6).

Taking Out the Trash

This crucial step requires going through your kitchen pantry, refrigerator, and snack drawers looking for items that feed disease. As you find them, throw them in the garbage bin. Here is a list of items that belong in the trash:

- White sugar, high-fructose corn syrup, and sugar substitutes (look for hidden sugars ending in "-ose" in ketchup, flavorings, and even bread)
- All boxed, packaged snacks and convenience foods (anything you'd call "junk food")
- Candy in solid or liquid form; that is, soda and juice, including diet drinks
- White flour — white bread, pasta, cookies, cake, bagels, muffins, and desserts
- Dairy — milk, creamers, cheese, and butter
- Alcohol — including wine and beer
- White rice and white potatoes
- Processed meats (bacon, sausage, salami, and deli meat), red meat (such as feedlot beef), and pork
- Trans fats and processed industrial oils like soybean oil, palm oil, and canola oil, which is made from GMO rapeseeds

As I've said, white sugar, candy, soda, juice, and white flour are on the trash list because these foods spike glucose, which leads to chronic insulin elevation, and chronic insulin elevation is a direct contributor to insulin resistance.

Please keep in mind that not all carbs are the enemy. Neither are all fats. When we start thinking about food quality, the breakdown of protein, carbs, and fats and even the calorie counts become irrelevant. Real food has a profound energy effect on the body that has to be experienced. It cannot be quantified in these oversimplified ways.

Here are some further explanations of this list.

Why Are Sugar Substitutes So Bad?

First, all synthetic sugar substitutes are nutritionally bankrupt. Second, they create cravings for energy-dense foods because the sweet taste perception is associated with the appetite regulators in the brain anticipating new calories.[2] The reward centers in our brain are strongly wired to seek out sugar as an energy source. Third, several commonly used sugar substitutes, such as saccharine and acesulfame, have been shown to produce cancer in animal studies.[3] Aspartame, a common sugar substitute in diet soda, is metabolized to formaldehyde — a potent brain poison. Fourth, sugar substitutes have a harmful effect on the gut microbiome (healthy bacteria in the colon; see chapter 10). You have about a hundred trillion *friendly* gut bacteria to feed and "care for": your inner garden. If you poison them, harmful bacteria can take over and control your food choices, increase cravings for the wrong foods, and increase the energy absorbed from food, thereby having a profound influence on health outcomes. Other than pure stevia leaf (an herbal product used as a sugar substitute for centuries in South America), on which the jury is still out, you should steer away from artificial sweeteners.

Why Is Dairy on the Trash List?

Cow's milk has the insulin-like growth factor 1 (IGF-1), which promotes rapid growth and can cause you to gain weight quickly. IGF-1 has also been associated with cancer-cell growth.[4] In addition, cow's milk is loaded with cow antigens (proteins that activate the immune system, resulting in inflammation), which may not be compatible with the human body. In addition, a main ingredient of cow's milk is *lactose* — a sugar that will definitely spike your blood glucose very quickly.

Modern dairy farm cows are typically kept pregnant year-round and milked twice a day. They are given artificial hormones to keep them in this condition and antibiotics to keep them from getting sick from their udders becoming infected.

The argument that drinking more milk provides calcium that will prevent osteoporosis is simply not valid. Osteoporosis is not a milk-deficiency condition. The United States has the highest incidence of osteoporosis in the civilized world, even though it has the highest consumption of milk and cheese. Cow's milk and products derived from it spike insulin and cause inflammation, which of course is bad news.[5]

And by the way, milk or cheese is an excellent delivery mechanism for cholesterol. Homogenizing milk creates particles that are small enough to penetrate the lining of the blood vessels and cause damage.

Holstein cows, which form the basis of modern industrialized dairy farming, have much higher levels of harmful and addictive A1 beta-casein than Jersey or Guernsey cows, the previous (though less-productive) industrial "cow of choice." We now know that A1 beta-casein strongly correlates with diabetes, as does the essential amino acid isoleucine found in milk.[6]

This is a good example of a food choice that causes hormonal imbalance as well as creating a toxic load.

Why Is Alcohol on the Trash List?

Alcohol is derived from carbohydrates that have been allowed to languish so that they start fermenting, as with beer and wine. A distilled spirit — also called a distilled liquor, including brandy, whiskey, rum, and vodka — is an alcoholic beverage that is obtained by distilling wine or some other previously fermented or brewed fruit, plant juice, or starch (such as various grains). Alcohol has almost twice the calorie content per gram of a carbohydrate. As alcohol cannot be excreted by the body, it must be metabolized by the liver. Whenever we ingest alcohol, the liver has to spend time away from fat burning to metabolize alcohol. The end products of alcohol metabolism stimulate the liver to produce more fatty acids and store them. In fact, you can induce a fatty liver with as little as three days of alcohol ingestion.

Even worse, some of the metabolites of alcohol are toxic for your hormonal balance. The bottom line is that alcohol is not a health food, and if you are trying to turbocharge your metabolism, alcohol does not belong on your menu at all. About 20 percent of Americans have a drinking problem. You cannot rationalize drinking for health reasons, not even red wine. In fact, most of the red wine produced in the United States is loaded with toxins like pesticides, mold toxins, and synthetic chemicals (to hasten the chemical reactions in order to maximize profits), as well as heavy metals and phthalates.[7] Ladies, all alcohol (including wine) is a strong risk factor for breast cancer.

As for resveratrol, the "magic ingredient" of red wine that has antiaging and anti-inflammatory effects, you would have to drink about 111 glasses of wine every day to get enough resveratrol shown in animal studies to be beneficial![8]

Why Is Red Meat on the Trash List?

Red meat contains *heme iron*, which is toxic to the pancreatic beta cells that produce insulin. Also, red meat (especially processed meat) contains nitrates, which reduce insulin secretion and impair glucose tolerance. To top that, environmental pollutants and toxicants are concentrated in the more fatty red meats.

Is All Fat Bad?

Saturated fat, especially from red meat, contributes to insulin resistance in several ways. Excessive consumption of saturated fat is believed to directly block the insulin receptors and the muscles, causing insulin resistance. It is also known to cause inflammation and oxidative stress. Unhealthy fats include margarine, commercial mayonnaise and salad dressings, hydrogenated and partially hydrogenated oils, and fried foods.

Good sources of fat include raw nuts (almonds, cashews, macadamia nuts, walnuts, pecans, pine nuts, and pistachios), seeds (sunflower, pumpkin, watermelon, flax, hemp, and chia), olives, coconuts, avocados, and wild-caught cold-water fish. These are healthier sources of fat, which can actually suppress appetite and promote Turbo Metabolism.

Don't All Fatty Foods Have Cholesterol?

Actually, cholesterol is only produced by animals that have a liver. The human liver produces about 800 mg of cholesterol a day, enough to cover your body's needs: to regenerate cell membranes, maintain brain function, and manufacture hormones. Most of the cholesterol in the body is recycled, so you actually do not need to take in any cholesterol at all. Cholesterol-rich foods include meat, eggs, and dairy, such as milk and cheese. If you eat more cholesterol-rich food, your liver tries to make less. If you eat less cholesterol-rich food, the liver makes more. Cholesterol is an important raw material that gets converted to vitamin D, steroid hormones (such as estrogen, progesterone, testosterone, and cortisol), and bile acids needed for digestion. Cholesterol is needed to construct the semipermeable membrane that surrounds the cells and to repair damaged endothelial cells, which line and protect the blood vessels. Cholesterol itself is not the culprit. The problem lies in an inability of the body to process cholesterol properly, or an inability of the body's antioxidant system to guard against oxidation of cholesterol. This is why a nutrient-dense plant-rich diet is so important.

Facts and Fallacies

- Alcohol, even in low doses, can cause breast cancer and birth defects.[9]

  ▌▌▌▌▌▌➡ Fact

  Technically, any alcohol at all is poisonous, even from mouthwash!

- Wine is a health food because it has resveratrol.

  ▌▌▌▌▌▌➡ Fallacy

  At one time, resveratrol, an ingredient in many wine products, was suggested to act as a protective agent against the carcinogenic effects of ethanol. The assumption was based on animal studies, which have shown that resveratrol above certain thresholds may reduce the incidence of tumors in several of the alcohol-related cancer sites (colon, liver, and female breast). However, the protective and health-promoting aspects of wine/resveratrol are highly exaggerated and simply not true.[10]

- French fries are 47 percent fat, and donuts 50 percent fat.

  IIII▬▶ Fact

  Fried foods have a lot more "dirty" fat from unhealthy, processed oils than we can even imagine! These create chronic inflammation and increase risk for cancer.[11]

- Avocados have lots of cholesterol.

  IIII▬▶ Fallacy

  Avocados do not have a liver, so they do not have any cholesterol! As I say, livers produce cholesterol as an important component of cells and for hormone production. Most of the cholesterol in the body is recycled, so we do not need to consume it at all.

Shopping for Health

After taking out the trash, your next step is to shop for foods that will keep you healthy. What you *include* in your diet is almost as important as what you *exclude*. Always choose real food — unprocessed whole foods or items made with ingredients that your body recognizes. If you can focus on food quality, you will never need to worry about counting calories or even about carbohydrates, fats, or proteins. Instead of counting calories, make the food that you eat really count.

I often run into my patients at my local grocery store, Sprouts, and they are always curious to find out what I am buying. First, you should choose a grocery store where you can see all the different sections from the front of the store and one that features fresh produce, as opposed to store layouts that confuse shoppers with thousands of packaged, processed items *labeled* as food. Nowadays, many small grocery stores, like Sprouts and Trader Joe's, as well as major supermarkets, such as Whole Foods, are introducing a wide array of organic produce — priced competitively — so it's easier to make the right choice.

Here are shopping lists for healthy Turbo Metabolism foods. Keep in mind that the produce and bulk aisles of the grocery store are where the health-promoting magic happens. Generally, the middle aisles of the supermarket are filled with unhealthy processed food and junk snacks, typically packaged in colorful boxes and plastic bags, replete with mascots of tigers, cheetahs, and other animals. Stay away from the middle aisles as much as possible!

Seeds, Grains, and Beans to Buy in Bulk

Seeds, grains, and beans are loaded with micronutrients and have a long shelf life. It's always a good idea to keep your pantry stocked with these superstars from the bulk section.

Please note that although many people substitute brown rice for white rice, brown rice can be contaminated with arsenic, so I recommend avoiding it.

Almonds, raw
Amaranth
Black beans
Black-eyed peas
Brazil nuts
Buckwheat
Chia seeds
Chickpeas (a.k.a. garbanzo beans)

Chocolate, dark (70 percent or higher cacao)
Cocoa powder
Flaxseeds
Kaniwa
Kidney beans
Lentils
Oat bran
Oats, steel-cut
Pinto beans
Pistachios
Pumpkin seeds
Quinoa
Sunflower seeds
Ten-bean mix for soup
Walnuts
Wild rice, black rice

Vegetables, Fruits, and Fresh Produce

Cruciferous vegetables are superfoods, loaded with antioxidants and cancer fighters; they are nature's "powerhouse" and the closest thing we have to a real "magic pill." See chapter 10 for more on superfoods. As often as possible, buy organic produce, especially for the "dirty dozen," or produce with the highest pesticide load (see chapter 9). Finally, there's nothing wrong with buying bagged prewashed greens, which are ready-to-use salad mixes or can be used as part of a smoothie.

Apples
Artichokes
Asparagus
Avocado (excellent source of healthy fats, protein,
    and fiber)

Baby greens or bagged mixed greens

Bananas

Beets, golden or red

Blueberries, blackberries, raspberries

Celery

Coconut (good plant source of healthy fats)

Cruciferous vegetables: arugula, bok choy, broccoli,
Brussels sprouts, cabbage, cauliflower, collard greens,
horseradish, mustard greens, radish, red cabbage,
Swiss chard, turnip greens, and watercress

Cucumbers

Garlic

Kale

Melons

Onions

Oranges

Peaches

Pears

Plums

Pomegranate

Shiitake mushrooms

Snap peas

Spinach

Summer squash

Sweet potatoes / yams

Tomatoes

Cooking Oils

Always use cooking oils sparingly. As for coconut oil, it contains medium-chain triglycerides, which may have some health

benefits, such as appetite suppression and brain health (and so could help treat Alzheimer's). However, at this point, we do not have adequate evidence for any of the health claims made about coconut oil.[12]

Extra-virgin olive oil (best for low-temperature cooking: under 350°F)
Avocado oil (better for high-temperature cooking)
Coconut oil (better for high-temperature cooking)

Poultry, Fish, and Eggs

Always eat animal proteins sparingly; try to limit them to 3 to 4 ounces, or 100 grams, no more than once or twice a week. That's a serving size about equal to the palm of your hand. Think of animal flesh as a condiment eaten for flavor or texture, or in the case of fish and eggs, as a source of healthy fat. Always buy wild fish to minimize exposure to harmful toxins.

Small wild fish, or SMASH, which is an acronym for salmon, mackerel, anchovies, sardines, halibut/ herring
Organic chicken (sparingly)
Organic eggs (sparingly)

Dairy Alternatives

Given the health hazards of cow's milk, use these nondairy milk substitutes.

Almond cheese
Almond milk
Almond milk creamer
Almond yogurt

Coconut milk
Dairy-free yogurt
Flax milk

Snacks, Spices, and Nutritional Supplements

This list includes recommended snacks, spices, and nutritional supplements (which are described in more detail in chapter 10).

Almond butter
Anti-inflammatory spices: turmeric, rosemary, ginger,
    cloves, cumin seeds, and black pepper
Protein bars (with minimal ingredients, all of which you
    can pronounce)
Raw chia seeds
Raw kale chips
Supplements: Omega-3 oils, vitamin B_{12}, vitamin D_3, raw
    coenzyme Q10
Vega One nutritional powder (pea protein)

Health and Beauty

Health and beauty products may contain a range of toxins and organic pollutants, and these affect health through skin exposure (for more on this, see chapter 9). Here are some recommended brands:

Dr. Bronner's castile soap
Dr. Bronner's toothpaste
Honest Company baby care products
JĀSÖN hair care products
Tom's of Maine deodorant
Tom's of Maine toothpaste

Facts and Fallacies

- The three top sources of vegetables in the United States are potato chips, French fries, and iceberg lettuce.

   Fact

  You can gain a great deal of weight on a vegan diet of French fries, potato chips, iceberg lettuce, and soda! Eat real food that your body recognizes.

- Pizza is classified as a vegetable by the USDA.

   Fact

  Thanks to the lobbying efforts of the dairy industry, which has an excess of cheese, pizza was classified by the US Congress as a vegetable (on the basis of having two teaspoons of tomato paste), so that the excess cheese could be sold to public schools (through the school lunch programs) and in the prison system in the form of pizza.

- The best-selling fruit in the United States and the world is apples.

   Fallacy

  In the United States, it's bananas; we eat twenty-four pounds of bananas a year per capita. Worldwide, it's mangoes.

- Watermelon can help with erectile dysfunction.

   Fact

Watermelon contains citrulline, which helps the release of nitric oxide. This dilates blood vessels so you can get more circulation to the parts that need it. Osama bin Laden reportedly ate a lot of watermelon to keep his many wives happy!

- Milk labeled as "2 percent" is actually 35 percent fat by calories.

  ∎∎∎∎▶ Fact

  In fact, 2 percent milk is 2 percent fat by weight, but 35 percent of its calories come from fat.

Deciphering Ingredient Labels

Ideally, you should buy very little boxed food; most of your food should be produce, which obviously does not have a nutrition label. However, if you do buy boxed food, such as cereals and snacks, you should not rely on front-of-box claims to determine how healthful they are. Here are five things to check and watch out for before you buy.

1. Check the number of ingredients and note the serving size.

Fewer ingredients are better, as are ingredients with understandable names. However, it is easy to be tricked into assuming that the amount listed of a certain ingredient is for the whole container, while it is really for only one serving. You need to multiply by the number of servings in a package to arrive at the true total amount.

2. Read beyond the first ingredient. Ingredients are listed in descending order by weight on food labels. This means a cereal claiming to be made of "whole grains" should list whole grains as the first ingredient. Did you know that a processed food can be labeled as "whole grain" even if it contains only 9 grams of whole grain per serving? Also, "whole grain" doesn't always mean high fiber, and starchy carbohydrates can pose serious problems for people with insulin resistance. Look for 100 percent whole-*kernel* grain. Then, read beyond the first ingredient, and if you see sugars, fats, and artificial flavors listed next, leave the box on the shelf.

3. Watch for sugars. Make sure the sugar content is less than 8 grams per serving. *And beware: Sugar may be listed under multiple names, such as maltose, brown sugar, caramel, and honey.* Some sugar-free, low-calorie, boxed cereals also contain artificial sweeteners, such as sucralose and acesulfame potassium, which are on the trash list.

4. Check the amount and source of fiber. Watch for added fiber in the form of *inulin* (not *insulin*), pea fiber, and bleached oat fiber, as these substances may not have the same health benefits as fiber from whole grains. Always check a cereal's label for added fibers; you want a cereal with at least 5 grams of intact fiber per serving.

5. Shelf placement makes a difference. It is sad but true that the most unhealthy, sugary, low-fiber, brightly packaged cereals are kept at children's eye level.

Track What You Eat and Be Flexible

The diet and other lifestyle changes recommended in this book are not rigid rules that hold for everyone.

The only way to know how *your* body is responding is to be in touch with it, to eat and live *mindfully* (see chapter 7). Closely monitoring how you feel — as well as your weight, waist circumference, blood pressure, and blood-glucose levels — will help you to fine-tune and personalize your own Turbo Metabolism program.

For example, while eating a whole-foods plant-based diet, some people notice that their blood-glucose levels spike after eating beans and legumes. The only way you will know if you are an individual with high carbohydrate sensitivity, even to complex carbohydrates, is to closely monitor your blood-glucose levels. The goal is to understand, respect, and leverage your own biochemical individuality rather than following the cookbook of any so-called expert (including myself). What works for others might not work for you.

The Glycemic Index

The glycemic index is a number assigned to foods based on how slowly or quickly those foods cause increases in blood-glucose levels. Also known as "blood sugar," blood-glucose levels above normal are toxic and can cause blindness, kidney failure, or increased cardiovascular risk. Foods low on the glycemic index (GI), that is, "slow-burning carbs," tend to release glucose slowly and steadily. Foods high on the glycemic index release glucose rapidly. Low-GI foods tend to foster weight loss, while foods high on the GI scale help with energy recovery after exercise, or they offset a low-sugar reaction. Long-distance runners might more easily burn off high-GI foods, while people with prediabetes or full-blown type 2 diabetes would need to concentrate on low-GI foods. Why? People with type 2 diabetes have insulin resistance, meaning their bodies are unable to handle a rapid spike in blood sugar. The slow and steady release of glucose in low-glycemic foods helps keep blood glucose under control.

Use the hierarchy of carbohydrates in table 3.3 to help you choose healthy carb options. Most of your carbohydrate intake should be level 1 nonstarchy vegetables, which you should try to maximize in terms of food volume. Beans and legumes (level 2) are rich sources of plant protein and fiber, but they can spike glucose levels in carbohydrate-sensitive individuals. Similarly, we should stick to low-glycemic fruits (level 3) that do not cause major blood-glucose spikes. Root vegetables (level 4), like carrots and beets, are loaded with nutrients — nature packed them with energy so that they can live underground through the winter — but they also tend to be rich in sugar, so you should be careful with your intake of these vegetables. Limit your intake of whole grains (level 5) and entirely eliminate foods containing white flour and/or white sugar (level 6). For a more complete list of specific foods and where they fall on the glycemic index, turn to appendix 4.

Table 3.3. Carbohydrates hierarchy

Level of Carbohydrates	Foods
Level 1 (maximize)	Deeply colored red, purple, orange, and green leafy vegetables
Level 2 (eat regularly)	Beans and other legumes

Level of Carbohydrates	Foods
Level 3 (eat selectively, 2–3 servings/day)	Fruit: stick to apples, pears, peaches, melons, berries
Level 4 (proceed with caution)	Root vegetables: potatoes, carrots, beets
Level 5 (limit)	Grains: stick to whole-kernel grains
Level 6 (eliminate)	White flour and sugar

Eliminate Allergens

The most common food allergies or intolerances are to shellfish, nuts, eggs, soy, gluten (from wheat, primarily), and dairy. One way to test your allergies to foods is to systematically eliminate suspected foods for six weeks. When culprit foods are eliminated, you might find that your skin appears clearer or migraine headaches or abdominal discomfort improves. If you want to try an elimination diet, first eliminate dairy and gluten for six weeks.

Up to one in ten people have some intolerance to gluten — the protein in wheat, oats, rye, and barley. Modern wheat has been cultivated to increase gluten to enhance the appearance and taste of processed baked pastries that we buy at the supermarket. Interestingly, the modern triticale wheat that is commonly consumed now has a lot more gluten and less micronutrient density than the original einkorn wheat discovered several thousand years ago. In short, we have modified wheat to maximize the appearance and shelf life of flour while creating unhealthy changes in it.

Again, there are no black-and-white "laws" etched in stone

for everyone. The only way to figure all this out is to pay close attention to what your body is trying to tell you. Increased heart rate, headaches, bloating, rashes, acne (or even redness of the face), energy level, and mental alertness while eating a suspect food can all provide a clue.

Mind Your Brain

Let's be very clear. You cannot fix your body until you fix your mind. Mind mastery is the key to your success.

You're here on Earth for a very specific purpose, and your life has tremendous value. You are a unique creation and were placed in the universe for that reason. Your body and mind comprise the vehicle that's going to take you through this journey, so you need to take really good care of it — starting now.

Your brain is essentially an organ of movement — it controls the physical movement of your body. It is also the organ of thought, perception, feeling, and action. Even though the physical brain is a mere three-pound mass of tissue (60 percent of it is fat), the software running on it — your beliefs, your attitudes, and your thoughts — constitute your conscious mind.

Achieving Turbo Metabolism involves reprogramming the mind to a "can do" attitude that overcomes the limiting beliefs and the "autopilot" settings that got you in trouble in the first place.

We all share the common goals of love and connection, of having beautiful experiences, and ultimately of having opportunities for growth and contribution.

Here's a little secret: The things that are good for your body are also good for your mind! (By the way, all those things are also good for your sex drive. Bonus!)

Following the taillights of societal and cultural norms is not going to work any longer in getting you to the destination.

The key to Turbo Metabolism is to adopt a new mind-set that helps you make the right choices, such as putting the right fuel into your body and saying no to the constant poisoning from addictive substances mislabeled as food, from addictive technological devices and gadgets, and from negative thoughts and attitudes. The dangers to your body are similar to the dangers to your brain; in fact, the risk factors for obesity and diabetes are the same ones that increase the risk for Alzheimer's and brain atrophy.

So, the journey to Turbo Metabolism starts with recognizing your unique and specific purpose in life (even if you don't know it yet), taking massive action to accomplish your goals, celebrating successes (even minor ones), and anticipating that slipups will happen from time to time and will require adjustments in your course of action.

Habit Hacking: Optimizing Your Settings

If information were the answer, we'd all be billionaires with perfect abs.
— Derek Sivers

While healthy eating, regular physical exercise, stress management, and getting enough sleep constitute advice that our grandparents might have provided, we all need the tools to move from knowing to *doing*, from thought to belief to massive action. Starting with the visualization of what the final goal looks like, this book intends to provide the nuts and bolts to manifest your vision into reality.

The strategy to learn new skills is summarized by the acronym FAST, which was developed by memory and learning coach Jim Kwik.[13] Here is my own paraphrasing of FAST:

F: Forget. As in, forget what you think you know. This is about starting with a clean slate, a childlike curiosity, "an empty cup."

A: Active. As in, be an active learner. Approach new concepts with full attention and the right attitude.

S: State. As in, be in the right physical and mental state, which optimizes learning and the adoption of new concepts. This helps move them from the conscious mind to the automatic, subconscious, habit mind.

T: Teach. As in, the best way to learn something really well is to teach it to someone else. You will master the concepts of Turbo Metabolism if you think about them with the intention of explaining them to everyone you know.

By understanding our universal human needs and by focusing on the end goal of living a life of meaning and purpose, of growth and contribution, we can move toward permanent behavior change. This is my mind-body approach to health transformation.

According to research, habits are a powerful tool in automating certain behaviors and actions so that they can be performed by the subconscious mind, like tying your shoelaces, brushing your teeth, driving to work, and remembering the lyrics of your favorite song. In fact, we are all creatures of routines and habits, and we become very adept at activities we do over and over again. We can complete 90 to 95 percent of our routine tasks throughout the day operating at the level of the subconscious mind.

If you have ever trained a puppy, or watched the behavior of dolphins at amusement park shows, you understand the process: a new habit is a conditioned (automatic) response that involves a cue (like a click or hand movement), an action (the dolphin jumps), and a reward (a small treat such as a dog biscuit or fish).

The same cue-action-reward sequence works with humans, too. For example, getting tired at 3:30 in the afternoon (cue) leads to grabbing a strong cup of coffee and a cookie (action), which creates a bump in energy (reward). Or on a typical Friday night (time cue), we feel the urge to go to a bar with friends (action), so we can relax while hanging out with them and drinking (reward).

The concept of *habit hacking* involves replacing a maladaptive or self-destructive action with a desirable one. Thus, we respond to the same cue by doing something different and then receiving a similarly satisfying reward. For instance, we could habit hack both examples above: when our energy sags at 3:30, we could go for a brisk walk instead of ingesting coffee and a cookie; on Friday evening, we could socialize and relax by playing basketball with friends or by dancing. The goal is to set up routines and habits to help us be successful.

Training New Habits

In the words of the Greek poet Archilochus, "We do not rise to the level of our expectations, we fall to the level of our training."

How long do you think it takes to form a habit? Many people cite twenty-one days, but that's not enough. This time frame actually came from a plastic surgeon who said it took his patients three weeks not to do a double take in the mirror post-surgery. In fact, the average time it takes to form a new habit, according to London College University, is sixty-six days.[14]

Thus, it's critically important to reset your world and to keep it reset for at least two months, so that healthy habits become the default choices. You will have the best chance for success if you follow these guidelines:

- Set your ultimate goal.
- Name an observable behavior that is in line with your mission.
- Be as specific as possible; choose actions you can measure or quantify.
- Focus on actions you can reasonably achieve.

Here are ten more things to keep in mind as you develop healthy habits and optimize your environment for success:

1. Substitute unhealthy actions with healthy actions: For the same cue or craving, replace an unhealthy food with a healthy one.

2. Schedule healthy habits and place reminders on your calendar. When will you stretch, move, express gratitude, or meditate?

3. Automate environments so that healthy choices are easy to make. For example, stock healthy snacks at home, in the office, and in the car. Keep gym clothes packed and ready to go. Also, did you know that using transparent glass bowls and plates increases our awareness of food quantities, helping us feel more satisfied with less food? Or that we eat 30 percent less if we use our nondominant hand? Try to work these tricks into your routine. This is the *most* important step. Automation leads to liberation from temptation!

4. Form a support group of family, friends, and coworkers who will help you stay on track, or quickly get you back on track, without judgment, guilt, or regret.

5. Identify cues and be aware of how you usually handle them, then see item 9.

6. Watch your language, and reword your options to limit
   bad choices. For example, ask yourself, "Would I prefer salad for lunch or dinner?" or "Would I rather exercise in the morning before work or in the evening
   after work?" Say to yourself, "Those cookies look really good, but they are not on my plan. I will have these
   nutritious almonds instead."

7. Piggyback on existing habits. For example, do ten
   push-ups every time you brush or floss your teeth. Or
   take a vitamin D supplement every morning with your
   smoothie.

8. Develop and identify your "keystone" habits. In an
   arch, a keystone is the piece at the top against which all
   others lean, and a keystone habit can help support all
   our other goals. A keystone habit can be anything, but
   often it's getting enough sleep and exercise. For you,
   it might be eating a good breakfast, getting a nice hug,
   having a good laugh, spending some time outdoors,
   hearing an inspiring piece of music. Even making the
   bed in the morning can be a keystone habit! When we
   lack our keystone, we may try to replace it with an unhealthy, ineffective alternative, like eating ice cream
   and cookies when we're tired. Keystone habits keep us
   on track with our goals.

9. Plan for success by considering "if/then" scenarios.
   For example, if you're going to a restaurant, review the
   menu online and know the best possible meal to order
   when you get there. If you are traveling and get hungry, then what will you eat? Pack healthy snacks so you
   can avoid all the unhealthy airport options. If you're
   going to a party, eat a healthy snack beforehand and
   plan to politely decline wine or dessert.

10. Reward yourself and celebrate your successes with healthy nonfood rewards when you achieve milestones. These rewards could be going for a massage or a spa treatment, or going to the movies or a concert. You might even shop for new clothes that fit better because your body is looking better.

RULES TO LIVE BY

- Mind and body are closely connected and constantly eavesdropping on each other.
- You cannot change your actions without changing your mind; adopt an abundance mind-set rather than a deprivation mind-set.
- You need a support team of uplifting people — your coaches, your cheerleaders, your tribe — to help you move forward.
- Take the tests listed in tables 3.1 and 3.2. Knowing your numbers is a valuable tool for improvement.
- Make a genuine commitment (not just a New Year's resolution!) to be healthy.
- Be sure to take out the trash. No junk in the fridge, no worries.
- Always take your "good stuff" shopping lists to the store with you.
- Superfoods, like broccoli and Brussels sprouts, are essential to a healthy diet.
- Think of food as fuel, not as an entertaining escape.
- Set up the right environment.
- Automation leads to liberation.

CHAPTER FOUR

Optimal Nutrition for Optimal Health

The best time to plant a tree was twenty years ago. The second best time is now.

— CHINESE PROVERB

Of all the strategies for improving health, wellness, and longevity — that is, overall health span — eating the right food is undeniably the most powerful. What goes in your mouth is the most profound way you interact with your environment. It is also one of the few behaviors that is 100 percent in your control.

In a nutshell, nutritional excellence is about maximizing the nutritional content of our food, while keeping the empty toxic calories from processed, manufactured, fake food to a minimum. We can do this by eating more plants, which are loaded with disease-fighting, health-promoting nutrients: green leafy vegetables; orange, yellow, purple, and red plants; beans; legumes; nuts and seeds; and some fruit. My friend Dr. Joel Fuhrman has famously dubbed this "GBOMBS," for greens, beans, onions, mushrooms, berries, and seeds.[1]

This chapter focuses on meal planning, meal timing, and meal frequency, and it urges you to cease thinking of food as entertainment or "comfort." Instead, I encourage you to shift to a whole-foods, nutrient-dense, plant-rich diet, one that incorporates at least forty different plant foods in your diet every week (six different whole plants a day, and three full dinner plates of vegetables). In addition, I encourage you to eat meat sparingly as a condiment. In this way, you will feed the mechanisms designed to keep you vibrant and strong. In other words, your goal is to eat lower on the food chain. The reward is an additional ten to twenty, or perhaps even thirty, years of vitality and productivity.

Avoid Processed Foods

As you add the right foods to your diet, you should also be eliminating the harmful substances marketed to all of us as "food." This includes most packaged, processed substances advertised on TV; sugar; saturated and trans fats; refined grains; most meat that is industrially raised in feedlots (especially red meat and processed meat); and dairy products.

Here's a good rule of thumb: If a corporation is spending billions of dollars to persuade you to buy something by advertising its taste, texture, or even its supposed health benefits, it probably belongs on your trash list. The fact of the matter is that we are constantly being bombarded by thousands of commercially motivated messages to acquire things that we do not need, to put things in our mouths that we should not, or to do things we really do not need to. Whether we like it or not, our decisions are being influenced by advertising all the time. It is up to us to decide which outside influence we will allow into our lives.

The problem with the "standard American diet" of processed, manufactured food is that it causes our blood-sugar level to spike. Repeated spikes in blood-glucose level lead to prolonged elevation of insulin levels, which in turn leads to insulin resistance.

In nature, sugar is "packaged with" fiber and water, which acts as a chaperone and regulates the release or availability of sugar. By refining sugar — that is, by separating it from its natural fiber, as by squeezing apples to make apple juice — we are essentially releasing a monster, a toxic and highly addictive, yet perfectly legal drug.

In addition, the unhealthy saturated and trans fats in processed food — and in fried or overcooked vegetarian food, for that matter — block the insulin receptors, thus causing our insulin to malfunction.

To make the situation even more complicated, 80 percent of processed foods originate from genetically modified seeds (mostly corn and soy, which are subsidized by taxpayer money), and then loaded with harmful pesticides, insecticides, and synthetic fertilizers. These unhealthy substances are then fed to cattle, pigs, and chickens to prepare them for slaughter quickly (see chapter 9). And then they all end up on our plate!

In addition, these animals are given antibiotics in their feed to make them gain weight more quickly. Did you know that almost 80 percent of the antibiotics we produce are used for animal feed? And these antibiotics added to animal feed increase their weight by 15 to 30 percent in the same amount of time with the same amount of food? This process is called "feedlot efficiency."[2]

Plants Provide Fiber and Plenty of Protein

A very important (and sorely neglected) component of our diet is *fiber*. Our Paleolithic ancestors ingested close to 100 grams of fiber every day, while our modern diet contains only 10 grams on average.[3] Briefly, an additional 14 grams of fiber cuts about 10 percent of our caloric intake because of the satiating effect of fiber. That means a high-fiber, plant-based diet can result in more satisfaction and satiety and less hunger. It also means we "take out the trash" more easily, thus preventing belly bloat and gas as well as colon cancer.

However, people sometimes become concerned about getting enough protein on a plant-based diet. I'm often asked, "I need protein, don't I? How do I get protein?" In fact, most people need between 60 and 100 grams of protein a day, depending on age and lifestyle. A sedentary, middle-aged adult needs less protein than a competitive athlete or bodybuilder actively working on building more muscle. But you don't need to eat red meat for protein. You can fulfill your protein needs from plant foods. There are plenty of elite athletes, even Olympic-level power lifters, who do not eat any meat! Also, like ordinary people, even athletes don't need nearly as much animal protein as many think. Of course, if you like the taste or texture, you can still have some animal protein, but please be mindful of its environmental impact and of the sacrifice of the animal.

Here are the best plant sources of protein:

Artichokes (also a great source of prebiotic fiber)
Beans, chickpeas, lentils
Black rice or wild rice
Broccoli
Buckwheat

Chia

Edamame (soybeans)

Hemp

Nuts (raw unsalted almonds, walnuts, pistachios), nut
    butters, and seeds

Peas

Quinoa

Spinach

Spirulina (highest protein density per calorie of all foods)

Tofu

Animal Products Can Be Part of the Plan

From a health standpoint, plants are a lot better for us to eat
than animals. Your goal should be to get at least 90 percent of
your energy intake from whole unprocessed plants. This means
we need to eat close to two pounds (or three full dinner plates)
of plant foods every day. As noted above, think about animal
flesh as a condiment for taste or texture.

As an example, a piece of lean organic chicken or turkey
(about three ounces, or the size of a deck of cards) daily can
provide an additional four hundred calories, which would equal
about 20 percent of a two-thousand-calorie diet; it also can provide an additional twenty-four grams of protein.

Oily fish can be an excellent source of essential fatty acids,
which are required for vital functions of the brain and heart.
They are called "essential" because our bodies cannot make
them, and they have to be supplied from our food. Healthy fats
can help with satiety as well. Again, make sure the fish is wild
caught to minimize the risk of contamination with industrial
pollutants such as mercury.

The Best Diet for Optimal Health

Regardless of protein and fiber needs, the million-dollar question remains: What diet is best for my overall health? The debate between the low-carb and the low-fat camps has been raging for fifty years, and either one can be good depending on the individual. Indeed, which is best probably changes over time even for the same individual.

There is no set answer for everyone. It depends on individual needs and health status, on activity level, genetics, and much more. Traditionally, from an Ayurvedic perspective, the type of food we eat depends on our unique mind-body constitution. In the future, as we move toward personalized medicine, nutritional genomics will help determine the optimal diet for each individual given their biochemical makeup.

I know of people who have done well with low–refined carb "paleo"-type diets, as long as they were getting enough plant power for fiber and disease-fighting phytochemicals from nonstarchy vegetables. Other people have done well on low-fat vegan-type diets. Again, the key is figuring out what works best for your unique mind-body constitution based on how it makes you feel and perform right now.

Mindfully eating different foods and noticing how they affect your energy level, hunger, satiety, and overall well-being is the key (see chapter 7). Your diet should provide steady levels of energy while eliminating cravings for junk food and energy-draining quick fixes. If you are eating what you think is a "healthy diet," but you are not feeling vibrant or the diet is too stressful for you, it probably will not end up serving you well. You are your own best guide.

In general, people with insulin resistance, prediabetes, or type 2 diabetes — this group comprises about half of the US population — tend to have higher carbohydrate sensitivity.[4] As a result, they would be better off adopting a low-glycemic, slow-carbohydrate diet with some healthy plant fats and satisfying (mostly plant) protein to maintain steady blood-glucose levels. By "slow-burning carbohydrates," I mean things like nonstarchy vegetables (greens and beans) that release energy (glucose) slowly. "Low glycemic" conveys the same idea.

On the other side of the spectrum, trained endurance athletes, such as triathlon participants, runners, and regular weight lifters, who are in the top 1 percent in terms of fitness, have optimized their metabolism to burn fat more effectively by having more lean muscle, rich in *mitochondria* — our wonderful fat-burning "furnaces," where the body burns fat and sugar to produce the energy it needs to keep us alive and well. These more-muscular individuals might do fine on a higher-fat diet and might even be better at handling a little more saturated fat. We will discuss mitochondria further in the discussion that follows because they are the key player in Turbo Metabolism.

Lately, interesting research has emerged about the ketogenic diet, which is a special high-fat, low-carbohydrate diet. Paradoxically, even though the diet is high in fat, it promotes fat loss in some people, but it can also cause worsening biochemical markers in others. The diet is called ketogenic because it produces ketones in the body (*keto* = ketone, *genic* = producing). Ketones are organic compounds that are produced when the body burns fat for energy, and they can be detected in the urine, blood, and breath. Usually the body uses carbohydrates (which get broken down to sugar) for its fuel, but because the ketogenic diet is very low in carbohydrates, fats become the primary fuel instead. Ketones are not dangerous in and of themselves, but diabetics need to be careful because having an excess of ketones can be very dangerous for them. Interestingly, the ketogenic diet helps to control seizures in some people with epilepsy. Typically, this diet is prescribed to epileptics by a physician and carefully monitored by a dietitian. Ketones are one of the more likely mechanisms of action of the diet, with higher ketone levels often leading to improved seizure control. However, there are many other theories for why the diet works for seizures.

The "ideal" diet is different from person to person and also can change over time for the same person. For example, in my travels, I have come across very fit people, such as the Sherpas in the Himalayas, who add yak butter to their tea (which might serve as a meal) and have tremendously steady energy levels; they do not have any issues with obesity or weight-related diseases. When these people move to the city and start working sedentary jobs, however, their requirements change.

Scientific studies on nutrition are really hard to conduct because it is almost impossible to describe and measure what someone is eating unless he or she is placed in a tightly controlled environment. Thus, many diet studies are based on self-reported food intake. Most of our conclusions about diet are based on observational studies, which cannot be stringently controlled, like placebo, double-blind, randomized controlled trials required for new medications.

The overarching evidence, however, suggests that three diets — Mediterranean, ancestral hunter-gatherer (or paleo), and vegan (or plant-based) — are the best for optimal health. What do all three have in common?

They all mandate eating nothing from the trash list! Instead, eat lots of real food: deeply colored plants, fresh local and seasonal vegetables, and some fruit, nuts, and seeds with lots of fiber and healthy fats. The goal is to get 80 to 90 percent of your energy intake from plant sources (vegan), and no more than 10 to 20 percent of your energy intake from animal sources. By eating this way, there is no need to worry about calories at all!

Figure 4.1 shows the similarities and differences among these three well-known diet regimens. Table 4.1 (on pages 86–89) also includes a few others: a mixed-balanced diet, which includes DASH (dietary approach to stop hypertension) and DPP (diabetes prevention program); low-carb, such as the Atkins diet; low-fat, such as the Ornish diet; and low-glycemic, such as the Zone or South Beach diet.

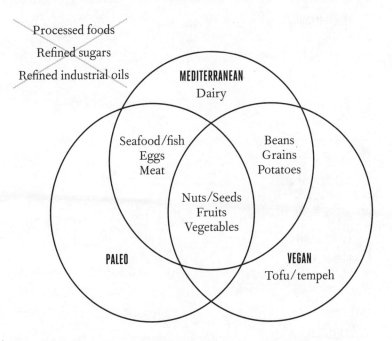

Figure 4.1. The similarities and differences among the Mediterranean, paleo, and vegan diets. All three diets agree that vegetables, fruits, nuts, and seeds are staple foods.

When comparing diets, focus on their commonalities to figure out what works best for you, rather than debating the minutia of their differences. The goal is to eat a diet as close as possible to the one that has evolved over the past several

Table 4.1. Fat, carbohydrate, and protein comparison of popular diets

Diet	Fat (% of calories)	Carbohydrates (% of calories)	Protein (% of calories)	
Mediterranean	30	50	20	
Paleo (ancestral hunter-gatherer)	25	50	25	
Vegan (exclusively plant-based)	14	66	20	
Mixed-balanced (DASH, DPP)	20	60	20	

millennia of human evolution: This is a nutrient-dense, plant-rich, high-fiber diet composed of real food that turns on the signals of healing, repair, and detoxification while optimizing hormonal balance.

Additional notes

- Emphasizes whole grains, beans, legumes, vegetables, nuts and seeds, seafood, olive oil, dairy, eggs, lean meat, and oily fish
- Emphasizes omega-3 fatty acids
- Doesn't aim for a specific goal for carbohydrates, protein, or fat

- Mostly plant diet
- 50 grams fiber per day

- Main goal is to increase nutrient density
- Higher in beans, lentils, legumes, nuts and seeds, tofu, quinoa, broccoli, and kale
- Plants are around 14% protein in calories
- Caution: supplement with vitamin B_{12}, omega-3, calcium, vitamin D, iron, and iodine

- Mostly plant-based diet
- Main focus is on nutrient density

Table 4.1. Fat, carbohydrate, and protein comparison of popular diets (*continued*)

Diet	Fat (% of calories)	Carbohydrates (% of calories)	Protein (% of calories)	
Low-carb (<45% carbs; Atkins)	30	40	30	
Low-fat (<20% fat; Ornish)	15	75	10	
Low-glycemic (Zone, South Beach)	30	40	30	

What about Meal Timing and Frequency?

It should be clear by now that eating a breakfast full of refined grains and sugar — such as toast, cereal, bagels, muffins, or croissants — spikes the blood sugar at the start of the day, leading to an insulin spike that will create hunger and cravings all day. Instead, for breakfast or earlier in the day, have more of your daily allowance of fatty foods, such as avocado, nuts, nut butters, seeds (such as pumpkin, sunflower, flax, or chia), and coconut flakes. This puts the body in a fat-burning mode. Having more starchy food, preferably complex "slow-burning carbs" after exercise, is advisable because that is when the muscles are more open and receptive to receive that nutrition and to grow.

Additional notes

- High protein content based on idea that it increases satiety
- Restriction in carbohydrates leads to calorie reduction

- Mostly vegetarian
- Best results for cardiovascular disease reversal

- Leafy greens
- Hierarchy of carbohydrates
- Healthy fats

As far as meal frequency goes, we used to think that people who maintain a healthy weight tend to eat three meals and two snacks in a day. They have frequent small feedings so the "gas tank" is never completely empty or more than three-quarters full.

We are now learning that keeping the feeding window short may be more advantageous. This means, say, eating between the hours of 9 AM and 5 PM (eight hours) and staying in the "fasting" state between the hours of 5 PM and 9 AM (sixteen hours). Many high performers skip breakfast or even eat just once a day. Here again, the trick is to find the strategy that works best for you.

RULES TO LIVE BY

- Eat real food.
- Focus on fiber.
- Nutrition quality is paramount.
- Feed your body the *right* nutrients.
- Healthy carbs, healthy protein, and healthy fat can make a meal nourishing and satisfying.
- Healthy fats maintain brain function, hormone production, and cell-membrane integrity.
- Ignore "My diet is best" arguments, and do what's best for *you* — every day eat a lot of produce, plus legumes, nuts, and seeds.
- If you eat animal products, consider the source and steer clear of feedlot meat.

CHAPTER FIVE

Water: The Stuff of Life

Water and air, the two essential fluids on which all life depends, have become global garbage cans.

— JACQUES-YVES COUSTEAU

It is no coincidence that two-thirds of the human body is composed of water, just as two-thirds of Earth is covered with water. In fact, the key to finding life in other parts of the universe is water because it is essential for life. The fact that Mars might have water is quite promising for the prospect of humans inhabiting Mars at some point in the future!

Less than 1 percent of Earth's water is actually potable.[1] The total amount of water on the planet has remained steady from the beginning of life. Earth's water has been continually recycled, but it has not been plundered and polluted by humans at the rate at which we have done so in the last century.

Water is a magical universal solvent that carries dissolved vitamins, minerals, and other nutrients, hormones, and neurotransmitters through the body.[2] Most biochemical reactions that make life possible take place in water. Water is a polar molecule and is highly cohesive. Polar means that it is electrically charged, and the electrical charge is different in different parts of the water molecule.

Cohesive means that the water molecules tend to stick to each other very well. Think about how a steady stream of water makes its way from deep underground to the top of an eight-hundred-foot-tall redwood tree. This cohesion is how it can form a smooth and continuous medium in the body for biochemical reactions. Body fluids connect us: The exchange of saliva and reproductive fluids leads to procreation. The cohesion and attraction of water is essential to life, and it has been throughout our creation. This cohesion manifests itself as the emotional bonding between people, and as such it underlies the experience of love. In all living things, water forms the cohesive liquid of the cell, whose vital life-supporting functions occur within the cell's cytoplasmic fluid.

We can survive without air for about three to four minutes; we can survive without water for about three to four days; and yet we can survive without food for up to forty days.

Among the many amazing properties of water, it is the only common substance that naturally occurs in liquid, gas, and solid forms.

Your Water Needs

Your body needs three to four liters of water a day (about a gallon) to function optimally. A good rule of thumb is that your daily water requirement (in ounces) equals about half your body weight (in pounds). For example, if you weigh two hundred pounds, you should drink one hundred ounces of water every day.[3] This includes water in coffee, tea, or any other fluids (except alcoholic drinks).

Meeting your daily water requirement can help you do all of the following:

- Feel satisfied and energetic while helping to prevent cravings for junk food
- Prevent constipation and headaches
- Maintain proper body temperature
- Flush out toxins from the bloodstream, the gut, and even the brain
- Cleanse the organs of excess sodium hidden in processed foods
- Improve skin complexion
- Help the digestive system
- Boost the immune system
- Prevent falls and other injuries
- Lubricate and cushion the joints
- Protect the spinal cord and other sensitive tissues inside
- Maintain our vital cell and DNA structure
- Optimize metabolic chemical reactions in the mitochondria that help us maintain our health and vitality
- Reduce fat stores

We are in fact dehydrated the moment we wake up because of water loss from breathing and sweating through the course of the night.[4] The first thing we should do when we wake up in the morning is to drink a liter of water to start the process of compensating for this overnight water loss and of cleansing as we start our day. Instead, we typically start with a cup of coffee, getting even further behind in our water deficit. I have nothing against good-quality coffee; I just think we should hydrate first. Coffee is mostly water, but because of its diuretic effect (meaning it makes us urinate), it could worsen your water deficit if you start drinking coffee in the morning without first compensating for the overnight water deficit by drinking a couple of glasses of water.

Have you ever felt dehydrated? Dehydration affects every part of the body, starting with the functioning of the brain. It affects mental clarity and energy levels, leading to fatigue and lethargy and worsening of response times and concentration.[5] Dehydration can affect our senses of sight, smell, and taste. It can affect skin tone and heart rate. It affects muscle tone and strength, making it much more likely for us to fall and get injured when we are dehydrated. Dehydration increases risk for urinary infections, constipation, and bowel obstruction.

A 5 percent decrease in our hydration level can drop our energy levels by as much as 25 to 35 percent.[6] Also, when we are dehydrated, we are at a much higher risk for injuries. Astonishingly, 75 percent of people worldwide are chronically dehydrated, and 37 percent of people mistake thirst for hunger.

Misinterpreting Thirst as Hunger

When we look back at the several millennia that we have inhabited this planet, the discovery that we could transport water in vessels such as clay pots has been rather recent. Prior to this discovery, our ancestors were meeting most of their water needs from food. Real, unprocessed whole food (such as fresh vegetables and fruit) comes prepackaged with lots of water. For example, a tomato or a cucumber is 90 percent water!

Thus, we have not really evolved to clearly know the difference between thirst and hunger, and we can easily mix up the two. This means that staying well hydrated helps us prevent overloading our bodies with food, especially with calorie-dense, nutrient-poor foods.

Drink Quality Water, Not Junk Water

Get in the habit of drinking the *right* amount of quality water. This is an inexpensive, quick, and simple shortcut to achieving the Turbo Metabolism solution of optimal health, vigor, and vitality.

However, not all water is the same. Just as beneficial nutrients are removed from modified or processed "junk foods" (and toxicants are often added), so water can be similarly modified and processed to become "junk water," in which minerals have been removed, and sugar, salt, and toxicants have been added.

With overuse of chemical fertilizers and pesticides, our groundwater has become more and more contaminated with these dangerous environmental toxicants.[7] With only about 1 percent of Earth's water being usable by humans, we should be protecting this precious resource a lot more than we are.

The quality of your water is as important as the quantity. Quality water should be free of environmental toxicants, such as pesticides, nitrates from fertilizers, prescription medications, lead, and arsenic, which are more and more commonly seeping into our groundwater. For the most part, the US municipal water supply is of very good quality. Of course, there can be stark exceptions, such as the lead-contamination crisis in Flint, Michigan, in 2015 (when, to cut costs, the government stopped adding an anticorrosive agent, and toxic lead from old pipes leached into the drinking-water supply). To check the quality of the water in your area, check for online resources and the Environmental Protection Agency website and safe drinking water hotline.[8]

Does Water Temperature Matter?

In Ayurveda, the recommendation is to have sips of lukewarm (or at least room-temperature) water through the course of a meal, and it's probably a good idea to drink a sizable glass of room-temperature water before eating a meal and to sip from it during the meal.

Why room temperature? All of your digestive enzymes work at body temperature, so ice water will make those conditions for digestion less than ideal. Ice water numbs our taste buds, which may be why we are encouraged to drink beer and soda ice-cold: It might be the only way to intentionally put these nutritionally bankrupt substances into our bodies. This does not mean that we should never enjoy ice cream or a nice cold orange, but just know that when you consume cold food or beverages, it might be reducing your digestive power.

Know Where Your Water Comes From

Sales of bottled water are on the rise, thanks to the slick marketing of this $8 billion industry about the perceived superiority and convenience of bottled water. Regardless of what the label on the bottle says, don't be misled by enticing promises and pictures of mountains.

In the United States, 47 percent of bottled water is tap water that's been purified, according to data from the Beverage Marketing Association, a trade group.[9]

The reality is that, for the most part, the US public water supply is much more closely regulated than bottled water, and it is the safest, most convenient, and most environmentally friendly option. Of course, this isn't always the case. In some parts of the world, bottled water might be necessary, and a can of soda may be easier to find and cheaper than clean tap water!

To end this chapter, I've provided a water glossary, which I have adapted from one created in 2012 by *Consumer Reports* magazine.[10]

Tap: Tap water refers to your community's public water source, or the municipal water supply. Nearly half of bottled waters use public water sources, which they then purify or distill (see below), but companies don't always like to advertise this fact. For instance, in 2007, Aquafina was forced to stop using the acronym "P.W.S." (for "public water source") on its label, which was considered misleading. Now labels say "purified drinking water," meaning they purify the same water you can get from your faucet.

Purified: Purifying water (from any source) means treating it to remove chemicals and pathogens, according to federal standards set by the US Pharmacopeia. There are many types of purification methods, such as distillation, deionization, and reverse osmosis. To qualify as "purified," bottled water must contain no more than ten parts per million of dissolved solids.

Distilled: Distilled water is boiled and then recondensed from the steam produced by boiling. Distillation kills microbes and removes minerals, which can give water a flat taste.

Spring: To qualify as "spring water," the water must come directly from the Earth, or from the underground aquifer that holds the water. The water can be collected from the spring itself, meaning from the water that flows naturally to the surface, or a borehole can be drilled to directly tap the underground aquifer that feeds the spring. Note that other natural-sounding terms like "glacier water" and "mountain water" are essentially meaningless, as there's no standard definition for those terms.

Artesian: This is another type of spring water, and it simply distinguishes that the water comes from a well that taps a confined aquifer.

Mineral: To qualify as "mineral spring water," it must be ground-water that naturally contains at least 250 parts per million of dissolved solids. These minerals and other trace elements can't be added later; they must be originally present in the water at the source.

Sparkling: Sparkling waters (like Perrier) must come from springs that are naturally carbonated. Typically, carbon dioxide is lost during treatment, so carbon dioxide can be added back, but only equal to what the water contains when it emerges from its source. Carbonated beverages like soda water and seltzer are considered soft drinks, since the water was never carbonated to begin with.

Facts and Fallacies

- Ice water is the best choice to help boost metabolism.

  ▮▮▮▮▶ Fallacy

  The ideal temperature for drinking water is room temperature. Water at room temperature keeps the digestive enzymes working optimally. Ice-cold water does not.

- All beverages are the same.

  ▮▮▮▮▶ Fallacy

  Caffeine-containing drinks, such as coffee, soda, and alcoholic beverages, ultimately cause dehydration because they are diuretic. The drink best suited to our biochemistry is pure water.

- Drinking soda or beer is a good way to conserve water.

  ∎∎∎∎➡ Fallacy

  About fifty gallons of water are required to produce one can of soda and about twenty gallons of water are needed to produce one can of beer. Industrial production of junk drinks is a highly wasteful process that puts pressures on clean water resources worldwide.

- Measurement is the only way to ensure adequate water intake.

  ∎∎∎∎➡ Fallacy

  A good rule of thumb is that when the urine is clear (only lightly straw-colored) and copious, your body is well hydrated.

- Blood is thicker than water.

  ∎∎∎∎➡ Fact

  Blood is thicker than water, but only a little bit, since it is 90 percent water!

- Earth is the only place in the universe with water.

  ∎∎∎∎➡ Fallacy

  Europa, Jupiter's moon, has a frozen fissure surface that hides a liquid ocean. It has more usable water than Earth. Europa also has sun exposure and organic matter that are the ingredients for life.

RULES TO LIVE BY

- Water should be the beverage of choice.
- Start hydrating first thing in the morning.
- Drink half your body weight in ounces.
- Room-temperature water is best.
- Drink room-temperature water before and during meals.
- Check the quality of your municipal water supply before wasting money on bottled water.

CHAPTER SIX

The Crucial Role of Exercise

My grandmother started walking five miles a day when she was sixty. She's ninety-seven now, and we don't know where the heck she is.

— Ellen DeGeneres

Here is the most important thing you need to know: People with more lean muscle mass are more energetic and burn more fat even at rest. Period. To burn more fat, you have to activate your muscles.

Have you ever wondered why some people seem to be naturally lean, while others seem to gain weight much more easily? Why is it that some of us need to be a lot more aware of our caloric intake than others? What if it's not as simple as calories in, calories out? In fact, the hormonal, epigenetic, and gut microbiome effects of what we eat are much more important than the mere calorie numbers. There is a lot more to the story than calories in, calories out. How else do you explain a 30 percent feedlot efficiency in animals given antibiotics and hormones while giving them the same amount of calories, fat, carbohydrates, and protein?

The amazing fact is that your body is a dynamic system constantly recalibrating itself. It's a defense mechanism inherited by humans over generations that protects us from shriveling away in a famine by cleverly storing energy during times of feast.

The Basics of Metabolism

A major part of the answer to these questions may lie in the way energy is produced and utilized by the body. In chapter 4, I mentioned mitochondria — the "spark plugs" in every cell of our body that carry the "spark of life." Mitochondria are the fat burners, the energy producers of the body. Mitochondria power everything in the body, so the more mitochondria we have, the more life we have every day!

To explain this phenomenon, let's start with some basic terminology:

Metabolism: This refers to the sum total of an organism's energy-producing and energy-utilizing reactions.

Total daily energy expenditure (TDEE): This is the total calories burned in a twenty-four-hour period.

Resting metabolic rate (RMR): This is the energy required just to stay alive. Typically, RMR equals up to 75 percent of our total daily energy expenditure (TDEE).

Activity thermogenesis (AT): This is structured exercise and spontaneous physical activity. AT usually equals 15 to around 30 percent of TDEE.

Nonexercise activity thermogenesis (NEAT): This is part of AT. It is the routine activity one does on an average day, such as fidgeting, standing, toe-tapping, dancing, shopping, and occupational moving.

Thermic effect of food (TEF): This is all the energy spent eating. It includes digestion, absorption, transport, metabolism, and storage of food. TEF equals 10 percent of TDEE. Complex, unprocessed carbohydrates from plants and high-quality protein have more of a thermic effect, meaning that more energy is consumed in their digestion.

Figure 6.1 illustrates the typical breakdown of the different components of total daily energy expenditure (TDEE) for an average adult: 70 percent is RMR, 20 percent is from AT, and 10 percent is TEF.

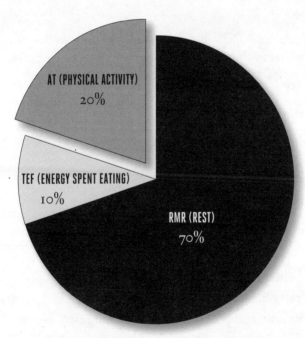

Figure 6.1. Total daily energy expenditure (TDEE) breakdown for an average adult

What Contributes to Our Resting Metabolic Rate?

If up to 70 percent of our TDEE is from our resting metabolic rate (RMR) — or the energy required just to stay alive, even if we were chained to a bed or in a prison cell — where is all this energy going? These life-sustaining functions are carried out by the vital organs: brain, heart, kidneys, liver, skeletal muscle, bone, skin, intestines, glands, and fat tissue. Table 6.1 lists each vital organ's percentage contribution to RMR. These are the bodily functions that are constantly running even when we sleep.

Table 6.1. Organ contributions to resting metabolic rate (RMR)

Organ	% of RMR
Skeletal (voluntary) muscle	22%
Liver	21%
Brain	20%
Bone, skin, intestines, glands	16%
Heart	9%
Kidneys	8%
Fat	4%

In the table, note that skeletal (voluntary) muscle is the most prominent contributor to resting metabolic rate, and it is also the only component that you can modify.

This identifies a key part of the Turbo Metabolism program, which can be simplified in three simple words: Activate

large muscles. All the muscles in your body have lots of mitochondria, which is where fat is burned for energy, and larger
muscles have more mitochondria.

Brown Fat vs. White Fat

Another factor in metabolism is fat, and we have two kinds.
Brown fat is healthy fat. It is *thermogenic*, meaning that it produces heat without shivering, thereby burning energy. How? It
generates heat by being rich in mitochondria. Eskimos, young
infants, and people living in cold climates have more brown
fat. As we get older, we replace some of our healthy heat-
producing brown fat with sinister white fat. Unhealthy belly
fat is white fat that produces inflammation and harmful messengers in the body, creating hormonal imbalance. Brown fat
burns energy at rest and is thus beneficial.

Eating an anti-inflammatory diet with turmeric and ginger
can potentially promote brown fat.[1] You might promote more
brown fat by keeping your room temperature in the sixties and
taking cold showers so the body is forced to burn more energy
to warm itself. Swimmers have more brown fat because swimming is a huge calorie burner — the body has to work extra
hard to maintain its temperature. Swimming is also an ideal mix
of aerobic and resistance exercise.

Increasing Muscle Mass with Regular Resistance Exercise

Of all the vital organs that are metabolically active at rest, skeletal muscle (voluntary muscle attached to bone) is the only one
that we can influence to some extent. This means that by gaining more muscle mass, we can burn more energy, even in our
idle resting state. This is because skeletal muscle is particularly

rich in mitochondria — those fat-burning minifurnaces within cells. Maintaining or increasing your muscle mass is a great investment; it is akin to having your money work for you even while you sleep! This is by far the most critical component to burning more fat and achieving Turbo Metabolism. So a significant portion of your exercise time should be spent doing some form of resistance or muscle-building exercises, even if that just means pushing your own body weight against gravity by doing push-ups, pull-ups, or squats.

The secret of fit athletes as well as regular people who look a lot younger than their years is that they have more skeletal muscle. If you want to lose weight and keep it off, build more muscle or at least keep the muscle you have! Mitochondria are your best friends; they are present in all the cells of your body but especially abundant in skeletal muscle. Which organs have the highest concentration of mitochondria? The brain, the retina of the eye, and the heart muscle. You cannot really modify the size of these, but you can definitely increase the amount of skeletal muscle in your body.

Skeletal muscle comprises about 40 percent of adult body weight. Your actual muscle mass is influenced by genetics, physical activity, nutrition, hormones, and disease. Although it is possible to build more muscle, it takes a lot of effort. But when you increase resistance exercise to load the muscles, you get benefits just for trying.

Skeletal muscles contain 50 to 75 percent of all the body's proteins. Protein synthesis and breakdown is what accounts for the energy burn in skeletal muscle. In fact, a four-pound increase in skeletal muscle mass can account for an extra fifty-calorie burn every day. And this may be all you need to maintain a healthy weight. Again, please keep in mind that it is hard work to build muscle, and it might take a year to gain four pounds of muscle weight. But this additional muscle is worth its weight in gold.

Regular resistance exercise should be an integral part of your exercise program to maintain and hopefully build skeletal muscle.

Muscle growth can occur by increasing: (1) the number of muscle cells, (2) muscle fiber diameter, and (3) muscle fiber length. However, cell number growth is limited to the prenatal and immediately postnatal period; you are born with, or soon reach, your full complement of muscle cells. Thus, growth is more likely to occur by either hypertrophy of the existing muscle fibers (by adding additional myofibrils that increase muscle mass) or by adding new *sarcomeres* (muscle cells) to the ends of the existing muscle fibers to increase their length. When we make the body work, it is forced to produce more lean muscle, rich in mitochondria to increase work capacity.

Muscles are very important. The only way the body builds more muscles is when it perceives the need because we are using them. In other words, "If you don't use it, you lose it."

Those who regularly engage in resistance exercise realize how difficult it is to build new muscle, but that's no excuse not to do it. The point isn't to become "muscle-bound" bodybuilders, but mostly to maintain the muscle mass we already have as we get older.

What Is Excess Postexercise Oxygen Consumption (EPOC)?

The benefits of exercise continue even after we stop due to *excess postexercise oxygen consumption*, or EPOC. For an hour or two after intense exercise, an energy burn of around 150 to 200 calories occurs. Thus, we can get a calorie burn advantage for a couple of hours after each period of exercise. How might you take advantage of this? If you do sixty minutes of exercise a day, you could split that hour into three or four installments of fifteen minutes. These quick bursts of resistance exercise (such as push-ups, pull-ups, or body-weight squats) would get the EPOC advantage after each burst of exercise! The higher the intensity of the workout, the higher the EPOC.

Fast-Twitch Muscles vs. Slow-Twitch Muscles

Skeletal muscles can be categorized into two types — *fast-twitch* and *slow-twitch* muscles.

Type 1 slow-twitch oxidative muscles: These are low force, low power, and low speed but high endurance. Marathon runners need this type of muscle. These muscle fibers are involved in walking and maintaining posture, such as neck, spine, and leg muscles; they are also called "couch potato fibers" because they are harder to grow. They are also smaller in size.

Type 2a fast-twitch oxidative muscles: These are high force, high power, and high speed but medium endurance; these muscles are developed from sprinting and weight lifting. Leg muscles have more type 1 and type 2a fibers.

Type 2b fast-twitch glycolytic muscles: These are high force, high power, and high speed but low endurance. Arm muscles have more type 2b fibers, which can be converted to type 2a fibers with regular resistance exercises, which build muscle endurance and muscles mass.

The proportions and types of muscle fibers vary greatly among adults; your muscles have all the different types of fibers, but the proportions vary and can be modified with exercise.

The new, popular periodization models of exercise training — which progress in intensity and workload and include light-, moderate-, and high-intensity training phases — satisfactorily overload the different muscle fiber types while also providing sufficient rest for protein synthesis to occur.[2]

How do you take advantage of this? Mix up activities. Alternate sprinting with jogging and incorporate resistance training in your workout to recruit all the diverse types of muscles.

Added bonus: When we engage in higher-intensity bursts of activity, such as sprinting or walking briskly up hills or running up stairs, we burn more white fat and leave healthy brown fat intact.

The Benefits of Regular Exercise

Many research studies provide substantial evidence for the benefits of regular, vigorous exercise.[3] To name a few, regular exercise:

- enhances emotional health
- improves memory and helps with nerve regeneration
- improves coordination and balance
- maintains brain volume
- produces more endorphins
- improves sleep patterns
- prevents dementia
- prevents and treats depression
- reduces stroke risk and improves stroke recovery
- prevents breast cancer, colon cancer, lung cancer, and uterine cancer

- prevents fatty liver disease
- decreases cholesterol levels
- prevents and reverses type 2 diabetes
- prevents congestive heart failure
- decreases blood-vessel inflammation
- decreases belly fat
- improves insulin sensitivity
- prevents age-related muscle atrophy and loss of strength
- prevents falls
- improves skin and wound healing
- prevents and treats high blood pressure
- improves peripheral artery disease
- prevents erectile dysfunction
- prevents and treats osteoporosis
- improves immune response
- maintains integrity of ligaments, tendons, and joints
- reduces arterial stiffness

Facts and Fallacies

- Over 50 percent of US adults engage in physical exercise at least three times a week.

  ⅠⅠⅠⅠⅠ➡ Fallacy

  Only 26 percent of us meet our exercise needs.

- The calories from a medium-size muffin can be burned by walking one mile.

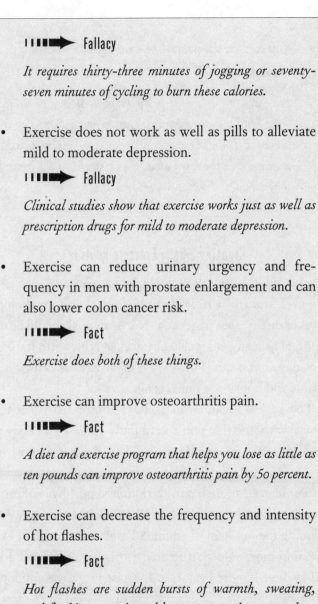

I I I I ➡ Fallacy

It requires thirty-three minutes of jogging or seventy-seven minutes of cycling to burn these calories.

- Exercise does not work as well as pills to alleviate mild to moderate depression.

  I I I I ➡ Fallacy

  Clinical studies show that exercise works just as well as prescription drugs for mild to moderate depression.

- Exercise can reduce urinary urgency and frequency in men with prostate enlargement and can also lower colon cancer risk.

  I I I I ➡ Fact

  Exercise does both of these things.

- Exercise can improve osteoarthritis pain.

  I I I I ➡ Fact

  A diet and exercise program that helps you lose as little as ten pounds can improve osteoarthritis pain by 50 percent.

- Exercise can decrease the frequency and intensity of hot flashes.

  I I I I ➡ Fact

  Hot flashes are sudden bursts of warmth, sweating, and flushing experienced by menopausal women; these symptoms seem to be less frequent and/or intense in women who exercise regularly.

- You can get six-pack abs by doing a lot of crunches.

  ⅠⅠⅠⅠ▪▪➡ Fallacy

  Six-pack abs are made in the kitchen. When we reduce our body fat percentage to about 10 percent, the definition of abdominal muscles starts to show automatically, starting with the linea alba, the vertical line separating the two sides of the abdominal muscles.

Creating a Daily Exercise Routine

Exercise might be the most powerful wonder medicine people have ever known. It treats both biological and psychological causes of disease (see pages 109–10). Your goal should be to incorporate as many enjoyable physical activities into the course of the day as you can. The body is made to be moving most of the time and not sitting much at all.

The key to creating an exercise routine is to engage in physical activities that you do regularly *because you enjoy them* — not because you *must* do them. Thus, the best exercise is the one that you will do every day.

Warning: Exercise has over a hundred health benefits in addition to calorie burn, and it may be the closest thing we have to finding the fountain of youth. Still, exercise is not an excuse for eating more. Most structured workouts only burn a hundred to three hundred calories. Exercise is not the antidote for a poor diet. Six-pack abs are primarily forged in the kitchen, not the gym. You will not improve your health until you combine both the right diet and healthy exercise in your daily routine.

The Minimum Foundation: Walking

Walking ten thousand steps a day — about five miles — is a reasonable goal for someone starting out as a "couch potato." Research shows that getting up to the ten-thousand-step mark has an incremental benefit. Beyond this amount, however, the benefit of walking does not increase that much. So ten thousand steps appears to be the sweet spot. Certainly the greatest increment in health benefit happens at the start — going from couch potato to regular walker.

Walking five miles a day (or 1.5 to 2 hours) may seem to be a large chunk of time for a busy individual. Walking can certainly be done in installments throughout the day. In fact, many of us already walk four to six thousand steps through the course of the day. It is important to keep in mind that before the advent of modern labor-saving machines, humans walked fifteen to twenty miles a day. Also, you can achieve the ten thousand steps in other ways, such as by changing your daily routine. Some ways to get more steps are to park farther away from your home and workplace, to use the stairs instead of the elevator, to walk while talking on the phone, and to engaging in more face-to-face meetings rather than sending emails.

Resistance Exercises

After you have established your walking routine, you absolutely have to start working on resistance exercises. The key to Turbo Metabolism is activating the muscles!

Just walking on the treadmill (or outside) is not going to get you to Turbo Metabolism.

You do not need to join a fancy gym or purchase expensive weight-lifting equipment. The most important resistance exercises are the ones that use the resistance of your own body weight and involve multiple muscle groups: the plank, push-up, pull-up or chin-up, squat, and lunge. These are simple body-weight movements that our ancestors have been doing for thousands of years in order to survive and not get eaten by a hungry predator. Most of the world still squats on the ground to poop, so being unable to get up from a squatting position would mean not being able to go to the bathroom!

The first step should be the *postural*, or *core*, muscles, which help us maintain our balance and strength. Core muscles include the big muscles of the lower back and abdominal muscles. Planks and balance exercises are excellent for strengthening the core. Interestingly, balance exercises are also very good for brain health, and loss of balance often precedes memory loss in Alzheimer's.[4] Planks are a very simple exercise in which you try to maintain a stable position with the weight of the body facing down, parallel to the floor, resting on the elbows and the tips of the feet while keeping the whole body parallel to the floor like a plank. Balance exercises involve balancing the weight on one foot at a time. Several yoga exercises accomplish this goal; sun salutations are excellent.

The next step is to start working on specific muscle groups. The big muscles of the body can be divided into pushing and pulling groups. Pushing muscles include the shoulders, chest, triceps, and the big muscles of the leg, such as the calves and the butt muscles — the *gluteus* and *quadriceps*. Pulling muscles include biceps, upper back, along with the leg muscles, gluteus, hamstrings, and quadriceps, which play a dual pushing-pulling role.

Resistance exercise is by far the most important exercise strategy to burn more fat and is far more important than counting how many calories you burn on the treadmill or exercise bike. The greater the percentage of lean mass or muscle you have, the more fat you burn. One more time: Muscle burns fat!

Developing Endurance

After you have practiced the basics, the next step is to work on endurance. Incorporate sprints into your routine of walking and resistance training. Called "circuit" or high-intensity interval training (HIIT), this process can enhance endurance. Keeping your heart rate up in the 140 to 170 range (depending on your endurance and age) is a measure of building endurance.

Endurance exercises build the capacity to maintain repeated muscle contractions over a longer duration of time. A rapid circuit of weight-bearing exercises, like push-ups and squats, interspersed with running or cycling, is a good way to build endurance. Sprinting uses up stored sugar in the muscle, and distance running burns both sugar and free fatty acids. When the muscles are used for exercise, they have wide-open channels to take in blood glucose like a super-absorbent sponge.

Once you start on endurance exercises, is it still necessary to continue walking ten thousand steps? At this point, it will be easy to get the baseline ten thousand steps throughout the course of the day. As you develop your muscle endurance, the focus should shift toward intensity, which becomes a higher priority than exercise duration.

A Four-Month Exercise Program

Here is a four-month exercise program that is suitable for all ages. However, it is particularly appropriate for adults who are largely sedentary and need to develop not only their muscles but new exercise habits. In a very gradual way, this program gets you fit by focusing on FIT, or frequency, intensity, and time.

The first goal is simply to prioritize physical activity in your life. You start doing that by developing a reliable routine, and then by steadily increasing the intensity and time of that routine. For four months, do the following:

1. **Frequency:** Establish a pattern of *frequent*, and ideally *daily*, exercise, of any type and length.
2. **Intensity:** Increase the *intensity* of each exercise session, so you work harder but not longer.
3. **Time:** Increase the *time* of each exercise session, so you start working both harder *and* longer.

Table 6.2 shows how I recommend doing this over a four-month time span. As with diet, no single schedule is appropriate for everyone. Consult with your physician and listen to your body to figure out what works for you. Also, keep track of your workouts, using an exercise log like the one in table 6.3. This is useful for following your progress and for sharing with your doctor.

Table 6.2. Sample four-month exercise program, with gradual progression

Phase	Goal	Target exercises	Postexercise activity
Phase 1 (days 1–30)	Building foundation	Walking: build up to 10,000 steps per day	Stretch afterward
Phase 2 (days 31–60)	Strengthening the core	Add body-weight exercises: push-ups, pull-ups, squats, planks, lunges	Stretch afterward

Phase	Goal	Target exercises	Postexercise activity
Phase 3 (days 61–90)	Strengthening specific muscles	Add shoulder, biceps, triceps, hamstring, quadriceps exercises	Stretch afterward
Phase 4 (days 91 onward)	Stamina/ endurance	Combine into a rapid circuit	Stretch afterward

Table 6.3. Sample exercise log

Date	Type of exercise/ activity	Effort (high, moderate, or light)	Total minutes	How I felt

How long you spend exercising is up to you. However, to start, aim for twenty to thirty minutes on most days, and steadily build to an hour. It's very important to listen to your body; let pain and exhaustion be your guide. It's also helpful to vary what you do. This reduces boredom and helps prevent injury. You might rotate between running, swimming, and biking, for instance, or perhaps emphasize lower-body exercises one day, and upper-body exercises the next.

Those who want or are ready for a more detailed and extensive exercise routine can turn to appendix 3, which incorporates weights and other specific exercises. In addition, *The Real Age Workout* by Dr. Michael Roizen is an excellent resource book on exercise.

The Four Biggest Exercise Errors

1. Thinking you can exercise your way to thinness (you can't). Food matters.
2. Overemphasizing exercise duration at the expense of exercise intensity. Think short bursts.
3. Training only aerobically instead of anaerobically. Always incorporate resistance exercises: They should take up at least half of your exercise time.
4. Letting "perfect" be the enemy of "good."

Special Tips for Better Training Habits

Be aware of common exercise pitfalls and take steps to develop optimal training habits:

*   Devote a specific time each day to your exercise routine. An appointment is easier to keep than random times. About 90 percent of people who exercise regularly do it in the morning.

- Start with short bouts of exercise. These will help ease you into a routine.
- Installments work, too: Do fifteen minutes of HIIT three times a day for even more benefit.
- Find a good training partner. While a training partner is not absolutely essential, support from a friend or family member will enhance your consistency.
- Listen to your body. Muscle soreness is common when initiating a new exercise program, but don't push through pain — work around it.

RULES TO LIVE BY

- Participating in some physical activity is better than doing nothing.
- Life is not a spectator sport!
- Sitting is the new smoking; stand and move whenever you can.
- Find movement in activities that bring you joy.
- Make an appointment with yourself for exercise.
- Work smart by doing multiple short spurts of higher intensity.
- Mix resistance exercise with walking, running, sprinting, cycling, or swimming.
- Muscle is your best friend in your quest for leanness.
- Six-pack abs are made in the kitchen. Fitness is achieved through physical activity.

CHAPTER SEVEN

Control Stress Before It Controls You

The only person you are destined to become is the person you decide to be.

— RALPH WALDO EMERSON

Happiness is when what you think, what you say, and what you do are all in harmony.

— GANDHI

At their very core, most physical problems — whether related to food addictions, alcohol, drugs, anxiety, or suffering in general — originate in the mind. Stress management is about reducing the "poison" that our mind sends to our body — mostly our own toxic reactions or negative thoughts about our environment. We can think about this dynamic as an "inside-out" process by reframing the picture, that is, by viewing our own conditioning about our relationship with the world around us. We can also think of it as an "outside-in" dynamic, by using strategies, such as relaxation and meditation techniques, to mitigate incoming stressors.

Developing your own system for stress management is the foundation for health because, whether you like it or not, what is outside is getting inside. Managing stress builds *emotional resilience*, which is the basis for adopting a lifestyle conducive to vibrant health.

Emotional Resilience and Willpower

Emotional resilience is the secret sauce of people who "get things done." It's about bouncing back from setbacks by being flexible, by bending rather than breaking or panicking. Resiliency is the capacity to recover from difficulties, the ability to spring back into shape, or the ability to withstand stress and catastrophe. Generally, resiliency improves with age. We get wiser as we are exposed to challenging situations and learn to solve problems. We can also deliberately enhance our resiliency by learning self-management skills and connecting with the meaning and purpose in our lives.

Whether participating in health-related behaviors or striving for success in relationships or at work, people who perpetually feel overwhelmed do less than their best; they just don't seem to have the willpower or skills to make the right choices. Emotional resilience is about mind mastery; it is about creating a feeling of fullness and abundance, of joy and balance. It's about exuberant energy and gusto to do our best and enjoy every moment to the fullest. It's about having the capacity to bounce back quickly from disappointment with poised equanimity. It's about creating the right perspective so that you can focus your energy on those things that are within your influence and not waste energy on those that are not. It is about understanding the simple fact that the only things within your control are what *you* think, feel, believe, and do and the kind of people and opportunities you attract. You have no control of what *other* people think, feel, believe, or do.

Enhancing willpower while developing skill power can lead to right choices even though you have easier alternatives. Willpower is like a battery that needs to be constantly recharged. Emotional resilience is the way to recharge the willpower battery, the foundation of building healthy eating and exercise habits. Why? Because it requires focus and attention to break old bad habits and build new and better ones.

So the next time you crave a food on your trash list, ask yourself: Am I really hungry? Or am I just bored, angry, lonely, or tired and misinterpreting those emotions as hunger?

The bio-psycho-social model of disease is all about how the outside gets inside, or how external circumstances get "under our skin." Quite literally.

Stress: Good and Bad

Feeling challenged to learn and grow in our day-to-day environment is essential for our well-being. *Stress*, however, may be simply defined as a state where the challenges in our life overwhelm our capacity to respond. Our bodies are designed to mount an amazing response to "fight-or-flight" situations, and this response typically works very well in life-threatening situations where all of our resources need to be mobilized instantaneously.

Throughout our evolution, this response would be what we needed to run away from a predator looking for lunch or if we were hunting another animal for our lunch. This response was designed to be quick and short-lived: it would last until the situation was over (we captured our lunch) or we were dead (and became lunch).

In reality, however, most of our day-to-day stress in modern times is psychosocial and non-life-threatening — yet our response is exactly the same as it would be if we were in a life-threatening situation. When we repeatedly or continually activate this fight-or-flight response, it keeps us in the "war/survival mode" and does not allow for repair in the "rest-and-digest" mode. It's akin to constantly having your foot on the gas pedal without giving the engine a chance to cool off. Or constantly keeping a rubber band stretched without giving it any chance to relax: The rubber band will wear out and break much faster.

Some psychosocial stressors are more harmful than our usual day-to-day irritations, and these are strongly correlated with serious harm to our physical health. Thus, these require even more awareness and the adoption of strategies to handle them, which this chapter discusses.

Published in 1967, the Holmes and Rahe Social Readjustment Rating Scale ranks stressors in terms of their likelihood to precede a serious medical illness.[1] The scale was designed by surveying five thousand people who had been recently diagnosed with a serious medical illness and asking them about stressful events over the prior two years. While much has changed in the fifty years since this scale was created (like inflation and gender roles), the scale itself is still valid.

Table 7.1. Holmes and Rahe Social Readjustment Rating Scale

Rank	Life event	Mean value
1	Death of spouse	100
2	Divorce	73
3	Marital separation	65
4	Jail term	63
5	Death of close family member	63
6	Personal injury or illness	53
7	Marriage	50
8	Fired at work	47
9	Marital reconciliation	45
10	Retirement	45
11	Change in health of family member	44
12	Pregnancy	40
13	Sex difficulties	39
14	Gain of new family member	39
15	Business readjustment	39
16	Change in financial state	38
17	Death of close friend	37
18	Change to different line of work	36
19	Change in number of arguments with spouse	35

Rank	Life event	Mean value
20	Mortgage over $10,000 [1967 dollars]	31
21	Foreclosure of mortgage or loan	30
22	Change in responsibilities at work	29
23	Son or daughter leaving home	29
24	Trouble with in-laws	29
25	Outstanding personal achievement	28
26	[Spouse] begins or stops work	26
27	Begin or end school	26
28	Change in living conditions	25
29	Revision of personal habits	24
30	Trouble with boss	23
31	Change in work hours or conditions	20
32	Change in residence	20
33	Change in schools	20
34	Change in recreation	19
35	Change in church activities	19
36	Change in social activities	18
37	Mortgage or loan less than $10,000 [1967 dollars]	17
38	Change in sleeping habits	16

Rank	Life event	Mean value
39	Change in number of family get-togethers	15
40	Change in eating habits	15
41	Vacation	13
42	Christmas	12
43	Minor violations of the law	11

Measure Your Personal Stress Score

To find out how stressful your life is right now, measure your personal stress score with the Social Readjustment Rating Scale. First, write down all the events from the list that have occurred to you in the past year, and add up the mean values. Compare your total score to this scale:

0–150	no significant life stress
151–199	mild life stress
200–299	moderate life stress
300+	major life stress

According to Holmes and Rahe, the higher the number you end up with, the greater your chance of developing a serious physical illness in the next two years. If your score falls between 150 and 300 points, the risk is 50 percent, and if your score is over 300 points, it's 80 percent.

The Harmful Effects of Perceived Stress

The bio-psycho-social model of health (sometimes called the "holistic model") posits that biological, mental/emotional, and social factors contribute to good — and bad — health. We can use this model to understand the harmful effect of prolonged or repeated modern-day stress on health.

Biological Effects of Stress

Stress is a condition of being overwhelmed and unable to cope with our circumstances. It is a perception of the mind. The part of the brain called the *hypothalamus* communicates our thoughts and feelings to the rest of the body. It does this through the autonomic (automatic) portion of the nervous system as well as its control of the endocrine (hormone) system. With stress perception, the sympathetic nervous system activates the fight-or-flight response within milliseconds. A little more gradually, the hypothalamus (through the pituitary) stimulates the adrenals to secrete cortisol, which eventually contributes to increased insulin resistance and belly fat (central adiposity).

Cortisol is great for short-term survival; it signals increases in hunger so that blood-glucose levels can be maximized, while simultaneously causing the organs and tissues to be more insulin resistant so that more glucose is available as ready fuel in the bloodstream. This can be life-saving in a short-term emergency situation, when the options are either staying alive or becoming someone's lunch, but most everyday modern stress is due to irritating psychosocial factors and not life-threatening situations.

Prolonged elevation of cortisol wreaks havoc on the body, causing weight gain, especially belly fat. It worsens insulin resistance as well as mobilizing energy by breaking down muscles. Cortisol and insulin are both weight-gain hormones when they remain high over the long term. High cortisol (promoting muscle breakdown) is associated with low testosterone (required for muscle maintenance and building).

The Nobel Prize–winning work of UCSF researchers Elizabeth Blackburn and colleagues shows us that chronic unmanaged stress affects us down to the DNA level by damaging *telomeres*: the protective end caps on DNA strands that help maintain the integrity of DNA. Throughout the course of our lives, cells are dividing, and our DNA holds the blueprint for the new cells that are produced. Over time, the ends of the DNA get "frayed" just like shoelaces wearing out at their tips. Telomeres, the protective end caps of DNA, are maintained by an enzyme called telomerase. UCSF researchers showed that stress management through mindfulness meditation can help maintain healthy levels of telomerase enzyme in the cells, thus protecting the DNA from damage. We are now learning that a plant-based diet, social support, and getting enough sleep can also contribute to telomerase function. Some herbal supplements are also being researched for their beneficial effect on telomerase. The more we can activate this telomerase enzyme, the better we're able to slow down the effects of debility and chronic disease, which we have come to accept as the normal effect of aging.

In fact, with high-fidelity cell replication and optimal telomerase function, we need not be aging at all!

Psychological Effects of Stress

The sensation of being constantly overwhelmed can leave us feeling hopeless and helpless, which, in turn, can lead to "willpower fatigue" — making wrong decisions when it comes to diet and exercise. When we feel chronically stressed, it becomes much more difficult to make the *right* choice. Making behavior changes can be difficult and the sensation of being out of control can be very challenging.

Social Effects of Stress

Loneliness is at the root of most self-destructive behavior. Social isolation — lack of family, friend, and/or community support — makes it much more difficult to maintain a rigorous schedule of self-care, health checkups, and/or commitment to medication (if necessary). The process of knowing what to do — and actually taking that knowledge to heart and putting it into action — requires emotional buy-in.

Behavior change involves getting knowledge across your emotional filter to take action. New awareness will give you a better perspective as you navigate through the spectrum of responses to changing your behavior: from conflict (opposition to changing habits), to compliance (begrudging partial agreement), to commitment (dedication to a more desirable, health-promoting way of life).

Thus, it is imperative to have a stress-management strategy for the non-life-threatening stressors that comprise the bulk of modern-day stress. You need to institute practices that help you activate the rest-and-digest relaxation response. This can serve as an antidote to the constant stress that you confront every day. It can be a quick reboot, a "minivacation" to a place of silence, peace, and bliss within all of us.

Tips for Managing Stress: An Outside-In Approach

Feeling overwhelmed? Stop and breathe. Observe your physical, mental, and psychological state. Rate the stress you feel on a scale of 1 to 10 (10 being the highest, that is, life-threatening). This kind of self-awareness will require your attention and practice.

- The gap between stimulus (stressor) and response is a magical moment that makes all the difference. By default, we are "wired" to react to stressors with a full-blown fight-or-flight response as though every stressor were life-threatening. In reality, almost all modern-day stressors are mild — 1, 2, or 3 on the scale.
- After ranking the stress, formulate a response on a scale of 1 to 10 as well. The idea is to match your response to the level of stress so as to avoid overreacting to relatively nonthreatening stressors.
- Imagine a "Stress-O-Meter" that gauges the severity of the stress. Count your breaths to ten. Then formulate a response that is proportionate to the stress.

The COOPS Model of Stress Management

The COOPS model of stress management, adapted from the work of Professor Robert Sapolsky at Stanford University, works well for most modern, everyday stressors — non-life-threatening irritations.[2] *COOPS* stands for control, outlets, optimism, predictability, and social support.

Control: Creating a perception of control can help us prepare when we know we will be in a stressful situation. For example, knowing that we have access to resources, such as pain medication, to help manage our pain can help make the pain more tolerable.

Outlets: Having multiple outlets — like outdoor activities, exercise, and music — can renew our strength to fight stress.

Optimism: Having meaning and purpose, such as from a religious faith or other spiritual source, can help us overcome adversity.

Predictability: Developing the ability to predict stressful events allows us to gear up for whatever comes our way. For example, knowing when our schedule will be exceptionally busy or when we might hit a traffic jam. Or knowing what the weather will be so we can dress accordingly or prepare by bringing sunscreen or an umbrella.

Social support: Having a team of close confidants with whom we can discuss anything without shame, judgment, or fear can help us get through almost any situation. This is the most critical component for all the above strategies.

Social Connections: Our Invisible Fabric of Support

Meaningful social connections, reliable allies in the journey of life, may be the strongest determinant of our health and longevity.[3] Recruiting support from someone who wants you to succeed with your mission is crucially important. Think about your spouse, friends, colleagues, and children. Ask for support and define precisely what support you will find helpful. Busy, busy, busy…this is how life seems to move for most of us.

We commute, work on the computer, check email, answer the phone, work on the computer, attend a meeting, and commute home, all the time mindlessly putting things in our mouth because they happen to be available, even if they are not really edible.

Although time may move quickly, there's this constant noise in our head, so we're not really present.

It's important that we build all our relationships, including our relationships with:

- others, such as family, friends, coworkers, and the world
- ourselves
- our spiritual life
- nature

Do you know about the Roseto effect? The Roseto effect is the phenomenon by which a close-knit community experiences a reduced rate of heart disease, and strong communities are known to have better health and longevity. The effect is named for Roseto, Pennsylvania.

From 1954 to 1961, Roseto had nearly no heart attacks for the otherwise high-risk group of men aged fifty-five to sixty-four, and men over sixty-five enjoyed a death rate of 1 percent, while the national average was 2 percent. Widowers also outnumbered widows.

In addition, these statistics were at odds with a number of other factors observed in the community. Roseto residents did not follow any of the other recommendations offered in this book: they smoked cigars, drank lots of wine, and ate an unhealthy diet heavy with meat and cheese, such as meatballs and sausages fried in lard. The men worked in the quarries, where they contracted illnesses from gases and dust. Astonishingly, Roseto also had no crime and very little poverty.

In 1961, a local physician discussed this with Dr. Stewart Wolf, then head of the department of medicine at the University of Oklahoma. Wolf attributed their lower heart-disease rate to lower stress because of strong social bonds. Wolf said, "The community was very cohesive. There was no keeping up with the Joneses....Everyone lived more or less alike."[4] Mutual respect defined relationships within families and within the community.

This could mean that meaningful social connections, the strength of our social networks, might trump all the other strategies toward achieving Turbo Metabolism!

Relationships constitute the single most important factor responsible for the survival of *Homo sapiens*. Evolutionarily speaking, humans absolutely need to belong. If we experience social ostracism or exclusion, the physical pain centers in our brain light up. The bare minimum is collegiality, but the real goal is camaraderie: kinship, support. Gallup polls show that close work friendships boost employee satisfaction by 50 percent, and people with a best friend at work are seven times more likely to engage fully in their work.

Identifying Your Support Team

Relationships are like precious gardens that need to be weeded, pruned, watered, and tended to every day. Like a beautiful orchard, they can be a source of respite from the onslaught of demands placed upon us. Mutually respectful and beneficial relationships are based on supporting, enriching, and energizing one another. There is no ego, no selfishness, no resentment or competition in relationships that last.

Why is developing and keeping meaningful relationships so difficult? Because relationships are messy. They can become strained over time, with conflicting interests and egos; they require constant nurturing and care. Holding on to grudges and anger is the single biggest factor suppressing our creativity, compassion, insight, and love. Focusing on the past — especially unpleasant memories that tend to reappear so easily from our archives — poisons our happiness in the present with ourselves and our relationships.

When our focus is on compassion, kinship, and kindness, on a foundation of gratitude and forgiveness, we can enrich everyone around us, and in turn, they enrich us. Gratitude is simply incompatible with dissatisfaction, which usually stems from fear, anger, and resentment. Gratitude practices are proven to have deep-rooted benefits to the person expressing gratitude. Forgiveness works much the same way: The benefit is primarily to the person who forgives, regardless of whether the person being forgiven is even aware of it. As a matter of fact, a key part of resiliency is letting go and forgiving ourselves and others.

According to a popular hypothesis, first proposed by British anthropologist Robin Dunbar, based on our average brain size, most humans can comfortably maintain about 150 social relationships in all. Of these 150, we might invite 50 to a dinner party at our home. Of the 50, about 15 people are the ones we communicate with on a regular basis, discussing our problems and joys. Of the 15, we probably have only 5 people with whom we can discuss anything on our mind without fear of being judged: these are the 5 people we could call in the middle of the night to bail us out of jail if we really needed to.[5]

We are the average of the five people we spend the most time with, so let's make our social network, our cheerleading team, our support team of our best fans as robust and uplifting as we can. This team will determine the narrative we hear every day about our own powers. It affects our state of engagement, energy, and passion, and it influences how we pursue the life we desire.

Building Resilience: Solve Problems and Express Gratitude

To build resilience and cope with the stress of difficult situations, there are two basic strategies or approaches: The first is to address the source of stress and attempt to solve the problem, and the other is to make a daily practice of expressing gratitude.

When you face a difficult situation, keep these suggestions in mind:

- Immediately stop overthinking, using distraction to avoid the problem, or denying the problem.
- Act to solve the problem. Even a small step helps: Write a list of possible solutions, or imagine what someone you respect would do.
- Know your triggers for stress and avoid them. For example, if you habitually check colleagues' schedules during lunch, don't. Or if you get Facebook depression, don't log on, and so on. Social comparison is a major source of modern-day stress.
- See the big picture, and put problems in perspective. Will whatever you are obsessively worrying about matter in a year...or on your deathbed?
- Show self-compassion. Treat yourself as you would your dearest friend.

The Practice of Gratitude

The second way to create resilience is by expressing gratitude. People who are consistently grateful have been found to develop a range of beneficial qualities:[6]

- They are happier, relatively speaking.
- They are more energetic.
- They are more hopeful.
- They report experiencing more frequent positive emotions.
- They also tend to be more helpful and empathic, more spiritual and religious, more forgiving, and less materialistic.

Step 1 of gratitude is savoring life's joys. People who are inclined to savor have been found to be more self-confident, extroverted, and gratified, and less hopeless and neurotic.[7] Savor the past by reminiscing about the good old days. Savor the present by wholly living it, being mindful of and relishing the present moment, and finding awe in small things. Savor the future by anticipating and fantasizing about upcoming positive events.

You also can express gratitude to those you appreciate. This isn't a necessary step, but research has shown that those who are appreciated get a big serotonin boost, plus the person giving the gratitude gets a boost, too.

Here's what the research says are the proven ways to incorporate gratitude into your life.

- Start or keep a gratitude journal. Write at least once per week, and perhaps change the theme each week.
- Display photos of who and what you feel grateful for, or include photos in your journal.
- Find a gratitude partner. Often we have a "venting partner." Why not have someone we can routinely share good news with?
- Express gratitude directly to the people you appreciate. Write a letter, send a note, or text or call the person.
- Incorporate gratitude into your spiritual practice.

Facts and Fallacies

- Occupational stress increases risk of cardiovascular death by 25 percent.

  I I I I ➡ Fallacy

  The risk is doubled.[8]

- Chronic and repetitive stress has effects on the immune system.

  I I I I ➡ Fact

  Unmanaged stress correlates with higher incidence of cancer.

Mindfulness

Managing stress requires being mindful about the here and now. The barrage of stimuli we endure every day from all our electronic gadgets is the antithesis of mindfulness. Technology is constantly distracting us with stimuli from outside our current time and place.

The next time you are walking in a park on a spectacular sunny day, note how many people are staring at their electronic devices, sending or receiving messages or checking social media, when they could be enjoying the present time and place. Our modern-day addiction to devices that are supposedly "connecting us" is actually taking us to a place other than the here and now. Why are we so afraid to observe our own thoughts that we constantly need to fill our mind-space with busywork?

The Seven Attitudes of Mindfulness

Here are seven attitudes that define or contribute to mindfulness: nonjudgment, patience, beginner's mind, trust, nonstriving, acceptance, and letting go.

Nonjudgment: Take the stance of an impartial witness to your own experience as it happens. This is the ideal "witness state" of a human being. Notice the stream of thoughts and judgments: "This thought is good/bad/neutral." Become aware without trying to stop the flow. The mind is constantly judging situations and people, but mindfulness means seeing things as they are without adding judgment.

Patience: Let things unfold in their own time, and practice patience with yourself. A child may try to help a butterfly emerge by breaking open a chrysalis, but this will likely harm or kill the butterfly. Why rush through some moments in order to get to other, "better" ones? Your life is what you experience in each moment. No particular experience is better or worse than another; only our judgments label them as such. Be completely open to each moment, accepting its fullness, knowing that, like the butterfly, things will emerge in their own time.

Beginner's mind: Too often we let our thinking and our beliefs about what we "know" stop us from seeing things as they really are. Cultivate a willingness to see everything as if for the first time. Be receptive to new possibilities. Don't get stuck in a rut of your own expertise. Recognize that each moment is unique and contains unique possibilities.

Try cultivating a beginner's mind with someone you know: Ask yourself if you are seeing this person with fresh eyes, as he or she really is. Ask yourself the same question with your problems, with the sky, with your dog, with the clerk in the corner shop.

Trust: Develop a basic trust in yourself and your feelings. Trust in your own authority and intuition, even if you make some "mistakes" along the way. Honor your feelings. Take responsibility for yourself and your own well-being.

Nonstriving: Practicing mindfulness means seeking no goal other than being who you already are. Pay attention to how you are right now, whatever that is. Just watch. The best way to achieve your own goals is to back off from striving and instead focus on carefully seeing and accepting things as they are, moment by moment. With patience and regular practice, movement toward your goal will happen by itself.

Acceptance: See things as they actually are in the present. If you have a headache, accept that you have a headache. We often waste a lot of time and energy denying what is fact. We try to force situations into how we would like them to be. This creates more tension and prevents positive change from occurring. Now is the only time we have for anything. You have to accept yourself as you are before you can really change.

Acceptance is not passive; it does not mean you have to like everything about yourself and abandon your principles and values. It does not mean that you should stop trying to break free of your own self-destructive habits or give up your desire to change and grow. Acceptance is a willingness to see things as they are. You are much more likely to know what to do and have an inner conviction to act when you have a clear picture of what is actually happening.

Letting go: Letting go is a way of letting things be, of accepting things as they are. Let things go and just watch. If you find it particularly difficult to let go of something because it has such a strong hold on your mind, you can direct your attention to what "holding on" feels like. Holding on is the opposite of letting go. Looking at the ways we hold on will show a lot about its opposite. You already know how to let go. Every night when we allow ourselves to fall asleep, we let go.

Meditation

Meditation might be a way for you to explore the fascinating world of the "inner-net" — the vast and intricate network of memories, thoughts, and experiences many times more powerful than your smartphone or laptop. Meditation is a way to instantly tap into the infinite source of peace that lies within you, to take a vacation to a place that is beyond the constraints of time and space, to dive beneath the turbulence at the surface to a deeper place of calmness and bliss.

Meditation is a wonderful tool that everyone should explore. It's an essential tool in your stress-management toolbox.

The ABCs (and Ds) of Meditation

Essentially, meditation is focusing your awareness on the present. How do you learn to meditate? It's as simple as learning the alphabet! Practice A, B, C, and D: anatomy, breathing, cycles, and distractions.

Anatomy: Adopt a comfortable sitting upright posture with the feet firmly planted on the ground and the spine erect.

Breathing: Bring your awareness to your breath. You do not need to change your breathing in any way; simply be aware of it. "Feelings come and go like clouds in a windy sky," states Thich Nhat Hanh, a Vietnamese Buddhist monk and peace activist. "Conscious breathing is my anchor."[9]

Cycles: Note the cyclical nature of breathing; be aware of each inhale and exhale. Some people notice that it is easier to concentrate while counting breaths.

Distractions: Distracting thoughts are an acceptable and welcome part of the process. Every time a thought arises, acknowledge and release it without judgment or shame.

Three Types of Meditation

There are three main forms of meditation: mindfulness meditation, concentration meditation, and expressive meditation.

Mindfulness Meditation

Mindfulness meditation is about moment-to-moment, nonjudgmental awareness. Martin Luther, the sixteenth-century

German professor and religious reformer, made this observation on wandering thoughts: "You can't stop the birds from flying back and forth over your head. But only let them fly. Don't let them nest in your hair."[10] Neuroplasticity research has shown that practicing mindfulness twenty minutes per day for eight weeks can lead to physical brain changes in many structures. The part of the brain called the amygdala (which triggers stress response) gets smaller, and the left prefrontal cortex (the location of executive decision making and positivity) gets larger. For some of us, mindfulness is a formal meditation practice, on a cushion, for forty-five minutes. For others, it's fleeting but meaningful moments. Meditators are able to attain both a profound state of physiological rest and a heightened state of awareness and alertness (as evidenced by brain activity).

Mindfulness meditation focuses your attention in the present moment, using your breath as an anchor. It's about being aware of what factors are in your control and what factors are not and removing as many stressors as we can without causing more anxiety. It's about handling challenges one at a time, without turning them into catastrophes or getting caught up in an eternal cycle of worry and regret. By reframing the picture, so to speak, we can get a better perspective on what is real and formulate a response to whatever stress life throws our way.

Concentration Meditation

Concentration meditation frequently uses a word or phrase, called a *mantra*, as the anchor. We build awareness of the present moment by returning our focus to a particular object (such as a flower or number), word, or phrase. Transcendental meditation is a popular form of concentration meditation introduced to the Western world by Maharishi Mahesh Yogi.

Using a unique phrase or word helps us redirect our awareness to a place of inner bliss whenever we want. Sitting in such awareness for as little as fifteen minutes a day can have profound calming and healing effects because it can allow us to "reboot and clear the cache." As Jiddu Krishnamurti said, "When the mind goes beyond the thought of the 'me,' the experiencer, the observer, the thinker, then there is a possibility of happiness which is incorruptible."[11]

Expressive Meditation

Expressive meditation focuses on becoming completely engrossed in whatever expressive activity we are engaged in. Examples include musicians, painters, dancers, or professional athletes when they are "in the zone." When I see maestros such as Carlos Santana or Ravi Shankar playing a beautiful piece of music, or athletes like LeBron James or Steph Curry playing sports, I think of the flow state that expressive meditation can get us in. Flow is the way people describe their mind when they want to pursue what they are doing for its own sake. This experience is not just for marathon runners or elite athletes and musicians, and it doesn't have to last for hours on end. It's simply that state where we are completely present for an activity that interests us. Flow is the thing we feel, or the place we're in, when the challenge of the situation is just slightly beyond our current capability.

Mindful Eating

As Dr. David Simon writes in his book *The Wisdom of Healing*, "According to Ayurveda, our ability to metabolize food is as important as what we choose to eat."[12] The ability to fully metabolize food and get energy from it is the basic difference between the living and the nonliving. If food is not completely transformed into its constituent energy and intelligence, healthy tissues cannot form and toxins accumulate. Thus, the way that we prepare food and our intentions and attention as we consume food are important aspects of its nourishing influence.

Other than breathing, eating food is the most profound way in which we interact with nature. David Simon outlines fourteen basic principles to follow in regard to the preparation and eating of a meal, which he refers to as Body Intelligence Techniques, or BITS. Below, I present twelve of his fourteen guidelines, along with some additional comments from me in square brackets.[13] As he says, "If you pay attention to these simple principles, you can help your system extract the highest levels of nourishment from everything you eat."

Body Intelligence Techniques (BITS)

1. **Eat in a settled environment.** If you are eating in cha-otic surroundings, you are metabolizing the chaos along with your food. Enjoy your meals in silence or with people that you love. [For instance, saying "grace" or a prayer to express gratitude before a meal can set the right tone and is a great tradition.]
2. **Never eat when upset.** The powerful emotional chemi-cals that are released after an argument do not con-tribute to optimal digestion. [These feelings can also undermine your attention on eating.]
3. **Always sit down to eat.** If you can't eat with your full attention on your food, wait until you can.
4. **Eat only when you feel hungry.** Your appetite is your best

friend when it comes to nutrition. The only way to be clear about the level of your appetite is to check in regularly with your bodily sensations and eat with awareness. When we overeat, it is usually because we are doing something else while we [are] taking our meal and therefore, eat past our satiety point without noticing it until we are stuffed.

5. **Reduce ice-cold food and drink.** For most of our evolutionary experience, we ate food at room temperature or hotter. All our digestive enzymes work best at body temperature. When we consume cold food or beverages, it is best to do so when our digestive power is at its strongest, that is, during the noon meal.

6. **Eat at a moderate pace.**

7. **Wait until one meal is digested before starting the next (2–6 hours).** [Allow the digestive system to recover from the stress of digestion before presenting it with more food to process.]

8. **Sip warm water with your meals.** This helps the digestive process work efficiently. By avoiding ice-cold drinks your digestive enzymes can function optimally.

9. **Eat freshly cooked meals.** The life force is greatest in meals prepared with fresh ingredients.

10. **Reduce raw foods.** Although there is no question that raw vegetables are richest in essential nutrients, if we cannot readily assimilate them, they are of little value. [Most vegetables release more nutrients and become more digestible if they are lightly cooked.

For this reason, uncooked vegetables, such as salad, are better digested with lunch.]

[. . .]

13. **Leave one-third to one-fourth of your stomach empty to aid digestion.** Leaving some space allows the churning process to optimize digestion. This state of fullness can be recognized when you feel satisfied from a meal without being stuffed.

14. **Sit quietly for a few minutes after your meal.** Eating is a sacred process. It is a magical transformation that allows for the energy of the universe to be transformed into the intelligence of your body. Savor the moments after a meal to appreciate the magic.

The Five Senses of Eating

Mindful eating, with full attention and presence, can be a total body experience. Honing your five senses to help you make the best food choices can also make eating a lot more enjoyable. This method works a lot better than portion control or calorie control, which is often destined to fail.

Sight: Unfortunately, most people eat with their eyes, not their stomachs, which is what happens when your eyes tell you there is still food left on your plate and you ignore the fact that your stomach is full. The next time you sit down to dinner and you've eaten half your meal, try closing your eyes and see if your stomach is still asking for more food. If you no longer feel hungry, save the rest of your meal for later.

Smell: Your sense of smell is strongest when you are the hungriest; you can smell food "from a mile away" and your mouth starts watering. To counteract this reaction, let your nose help tell you when you are full: If you smell your food partway through your meal, and your mouth is no longer watering, it may be time to stop eating.

Touch: How food feels in your mouth is a good indication of a healthier choice. Pick foods that are fibrous and take a while to chew, not the ones that simply "melt in your mouth." These foods will take longer to digest and give you a full feeling for a longer time.

Hearing: Studies have shown that people who listen to loud music while eating tend to eat longer and consume more food. Likewise, people who listen to loud music while drinking tend to finish drinks faster and order more of them.[14] While dinner music may seem pleasant, try eating in silence or engage in casual conversation with a companion, and let your mind and body focus on the meal.

Taste: This may seem like the most obvious sense when it comes to eating, but taste may also take the most time to train (or retrain). You can train your taste buds to prefer food a certain way — with a lot of sugar or salt, for example. It may take some time, but you can train your taste buds to prefer low-sugar or low-salt foods. Start by slowly reducing the amount of salt you cook with, as well as limiting processed foods containing sodium. Over time, you will not even notice the lower sodium content, and you will become more wary of highly salted food.

Training Your Senses: The STOP Method

Here's a practice you can do anywhere at any time simply by remembering the acronym STOP, originally created by Dr. Elisha Goldstein.[15]

S – Stop what you are doing.

T – Take a breath. Pay attention as your breath slowly and naturally moves in and out of your body. To help focus, you could also say to yourself "in" as you inhale and "out" as you exhale.

O – Observe your body, emotions, and mind. Examine your posture: Is it hunched over? Do you notice any tension or tightness? What emotions are you experiencing? These are sometimes harder to self-assess. Do you notice frustration, irritation, calmness, fatigue? Excitement, sadness, or joy? Finally, check in with your mind — is it busy or calm? You may even catch your mind talking or processing images as you pay attention to it.

P – Proceed with what is most important right now. Prioritize and refocus your attention to where it is most needed.

Know Your Type and Relieve Stress from the Inside Out

Everyone may be unique, but people also adopt certain "typical" or habitual responses to problems and stress. That is, people can reflect types, and knowing yours will offer clues about how to relieve stress. Take an "inside-out" approach and reflect on how you view the external world.

For instance, do you tend to adopt a "victim mentality," where you blame others rather than looking at your own role in your current situation? Or do you prefer to be in "driver mode," which constantly wants to be dominant or in charge? Are you a type A personality — someone who's often over-achieving, time-pressured, competitive, impatient, and hostile — or a type B, someone who usually prefers playing over winning, and creating more than achieving?

Type A personality traits, especially cynical hostility, are particularly associated with cardiometabolic diseases.[16] Sometimes, actively reframing the picture can lead to a better perspective.

Cardiologists Meyer Friedman and Ray Rosenman coined the term *type A personality* in the 1960s after spending a fortune reupholstering the chairs in their waiting rooms.[17] One day, a new upholsterer came in to examine the wear and tear, took one look at the chairs, and exclaimed: "What the hell is wrong with your patients? People don't wear out chairs this way." The cardiologists realized that their heart patients habitually sat on the edges of their seats, fidgeting and clawing away at the armrests.

What they found was that there is a very strong correlation between type A personalities and heart disease. Certain high-pressure professions, like lawyers and doctors, show this. For instance, in one study, male physicians who had measured high on hostility scores twenty-five years before had four times higher risk of coronary artery disease and six times higher risk of mortality.[18]

The hallmark of cynical hostility is the absence of trust in the goodness of others, and people who exhibit this tend to agree with statements like: "Most people make friends because friends are likely to be useful to them," and "I have frequently worked under people who have things arranged so they can get credit for good work but are able to pass off mistakes onto those under them."

Ultimately, the most effective ways to increase happiness, optimism, and resilience depend on each unique individual and each particular situation. Paths to greater wellness are varied. It's a lot like musical tastes. Different people may prefer Beethoven, Bach, the Beach Boys, Beyoncé, or Bobby Lewis, but the joy each person feels while listening is the same. Be sure to pursue the strategies that resonate best with you.

Throughout this chapter, you may find that you are more interested in some stress-relief approaches than others. Practice these, and don't feel you have to magically adopt every new habit to succeed. Hopefully, at least one or two will resonate, and you'll think, "Yeah, I could benefit from doing that." Choose to increase the actions that you're already doing — increasing frequency, being more consistent — or as an experiment, start something new that you wouldn't naturally gravitate toward and see if it helps.

CASE STUDY: VIJAY

Vijay, a fifty-one-year-old software executive, was diagnosed with type 2 diabetes and put on Metformin and other medications. He had tried various diet plans and was told that he would be on Metformin for his whole life and eventually insulin. Then he had a tragedy in his family that broke him completely. After attending my program, he found new energy and a different perspective on lifestyle, diet, and exercise. He concluded that emotional resilience was the most important aspect of his treatment. He realized that he had been using food as therapy.

When he discovered yoga and meditation, he was able to get back to eating mindfully. His HbA1c improved from 8.5 percent to 7.3 percent; his belly dimension decreased by 2.5 inches; and his LDL/HDL also improved. He realized that type 2 diabetes is reversible, and he is grateful to have found renewed joy in life.

CASE STUDY: VICTORIA

Victoria, a forty-six-year-old business owner, gained thirty-five pounds after a tragic accident took her daughter's life. She found herself eating to help relieve her sorrow and loneliness. After entering my program, she regained her composure. She returned to eating for nourishment and satiety. Victoria also recognized that she needed to work on her spiritual and emotional strength to help her cope with her personal tragedy. She joined a support group to start her healing process.

In two months she lost twenty pounds and regained her confidence. Though she continues to have bad days, Victoria realizes that food can give her energy but will not relieve her pain. She participates in mindful breathing exercises every day and tries to get plenty of sleep, while she draws strength from her support group and her supportive group of friends.

RULES TO LIVE BY

- There is a profound mind-body connection.
- Emotional health is the key to putting knowledge into practice.
- Stress is a normal part of modern life.
- Stress management is an essential skill; use your energy wisely.
- Choosing your responses to stress makes all the difference.
- Our perception of control and predictability makes unpleasant situations more tolerable.
- Music, art, meditation, and deep connections with family and friends are possible outlets for alleviating stress.
- Optimism is a positive trait that can be developed.
- Meaning, purpose, and joy sustain us.
- Quiet times help us reconnect with our personal power; take breaks from technology.
- Reframe the picture if your current frame is not working.
- Social connections are a major factor in our ability to keep good habits.
- Forgiveness and gratitude are powerful tools.
- Be here now.
- A proven way to increase your resilience is to commit to your goals.

CHAPTER EIGHT

Sleep: A Vital Component of Health

Dreaming, after all, is a form of planning.
— GLORIA STEINEM

*Getting enough sleep doesn't mean that you are giving up your goals
or your desire to achieve and succeed — on the contrary, it makes you
more effective....It's a performance enhancer.*
— ARIANNA HUFFINGTON

What do basketball legend LeBron James, journalist and entrepreneur Arianna Huffington, and Bollywood superstar Aamir Khan have in common, other than exceptional talent and an impeccable work ethic? They all prioritize sleep over most other activities! They all realize that getting enough sleep — both in quality and quantity — is the secret to achieving the highest level of performance. If it were not that important, why would humans have evolved to spend one-third of our lives sleeping?

Consider the following:

- Basketball and tennis players get a 42 percent boost in sports performance and accuracy by getting enough sleep.
- Sleep deprivation was a factor in the *Valdez* oil spill, the *Challenger* space shuttle disaster, and the nuclear accident on Three Mile Island.
- One hundred thousand motor vehicle accidents attributable to sleep deprivation are reported in the United States every year, resulting in seventy-six thousand injuries and fifteen thousand deaths. That is the equivalent of fifty airplane crashes every year with no survivors!
- The US military correlates sleep with significant improvements in accuracy and decision making.
- Twenty-four hours of sleep deprivation impairs driving to the same extent as being legally drunk.

And most impressive, a twenty-to-thirty-minute power nap improves alertness by 100 percent. This is why pro athletes and ace performers often take naps before a big game or performance, and so should you!

Basketball legend LeBron James has said that he prioritizes getting twelve hours of sleep every night, and many of his NBA colleagues take a power nap before practice or a big game. The military has studied this in great detail and has shown that there is a 25 percent reduction in cognitive ability with every successive twenty-four hours a person is awake.

Contrary to popular belief, sleep is not just passive rest; it's a complex active phenomenon involving physical, mental, and psychological systems working in perfect synchrony. It's a "force multiplier" that can make us bigger, better, faster, and stronger. Getting enough quality sleep might be the most important component of the Turbo Metabolism strategy because it affects our appetite, food choices, metabolism, and weight, and it influences our memory and focus, energy levels, and immune system.

If that's so, then why is sleep the first thing we compromise whenever we can, whether to celebrate and "party all night" or when we encounter time pressure? Nowadays, working efficiently is often equated with "working 24/7," "pulling all-nighters," and "hustling." In the early twentieth century, people slept on average nine hours a night, and most people still require about seven to nine hours of sleep. This has not changed even though we are living in a world of nonstop stimulation from our electronic devices and gadgets. Americans now sleep on average only six to seven hours a night.[1]

The nineteenth-century Industrial Revolution meant assembly lines could run twenty-four hours a day, and along with assembly lines came the idea of shift work. Today, our constant connectivity, from the internet and smartphones, has essentially added a thirteenth month of work. Did you know that night-shift workers have a much higher risk of health problems, including breast cancer?[2]

How much sleep do you need? The amount that you need is unique to you, and you cannot "learn" to function with less than your ideal amount. It is not about what time you wake up, but how you feel when you do. So, the right sleep duration for you should allow you to:

- easily get out of bed, refreshed
- not feel sleepy during the daytime
- easily concentrate and think clearly
- maintain a generally good mood

Sleep Deprivation and Chronic Disease

A dose-response relationship exists between short sleep duration and metabolic syndrome (see chapter 1). Those who
sleep less than five hours a day have 1.5 higher odds of developing metabolic syndrome.[3] Short sleep duration is also directly correlated with being overweight, obesity, and diabetes.[4]
This correlation is commonly observed in people who work the
night shift or otherwise compromise on sleep and quickly gain
weight and become insulin resistant, sometimes in as little as
three days! That's right, working the night shift can make you
fat, tired, hungry, and diabetic!

We know that lack of sleep increases ghrelin, the hunger
hormone, along with decreasing leptin, the satiety hormone,
thus signaling us to be hungrier and to store energy as fat.
Lack of sleep also increases the secretion of cortisol, the stress
hormone (see chapter 7), by up to 25 percent, thus promoting
hunger and insulin resistance.[5] This is nature's elegant way of
trying to protect us. As lack of sleep is a major stressor, the
body is acting out of self-preservation to increase appetite and
produce cravings for calorie-dense (fatty, sugary) foods to
maintain the energy supply. To top that, sleep deprivation decreases blood flow to the prefrontal cortex: the part of the brain
that helps us make rational decisions.

Sleep deprivation is also associated with decreased immunity and memory difficulties. In fact, studies have shown that
sleeping seven hours instead of eight triples your risk for catch-
ing a cold.[6] Sleep deprivation, whether from insomnia or lack
of opportunity, costs the US economy $100 billion a year when
you factor in lost productivity, medical expenses, sick leave,
and property and environmental damage.

In other words, sleep affects many aspects of our physical health. A short list of the main functions include the following:

- Cellular growth and repair
- Hormone production
- Inflammation reduction
- Endogenous antioxidant defense
- Energy replenishment
- Emotional and mental restoration
- Neuroplasticity improvement
- Memory formation and consolidation

Melatonin and Serotonin

Melatonin, the hormone produced in the pineal gland and in response to darkness, is the normal signal for us to fall asleep. In the evening hours, the more we are exposed to light from artificial sources like television, laptop screens, LED bulbs, and smartphones, the less melatonin the body is able to produce to put us into a restful state. When melatonin is low, cortisol (the stress hormone) is high, which also makes sleep difficult.

Serotonin, another hormone that regulates sleep and calms us down, is also light sensitive and directly related to melatonin. In fact, melatonin is produced from serotonin. As darkness approaches, the body's serotonin levels rise and melatonin is released to start the natural sleep cycle. A deficiency in serotonin due to exposure to bright, artificial light at night will affect the production of melatonin, and you will not sleep well. Interestingly, a lack of serotonin also makes us depressed! Melatonin is a magical hormone; it not only regulates your natural sleep pattern, it reduces stress as well. Melatonin is also an antioxidant, which means it slows down the aging process, decreases cholesterol, and generally makes you feel better!

Sleep deprivation is probably the single most important contributor to unhealthy lifestyle choices that lead to disease. When we "rest and digest," we repair damage to the body before it becomes irreversible. Cleaning crews of gut bacteria (see chapter 10) come in to detoxify the system much like the janitorial crew in an office building. Memory is consolidated and the immune system is "recharged." The immune system serves as a surveillance mechanism — for both outside invaders and "rogue" cancer cells — to seek out and destroy them before they can even be detected.

As with unmanaged stress, sleep deprivation is tolerated in the short term by the activation of the fight-or-flight survival mechanisms, which amounts to burning the candle at both ends. This may be one of the reasons why, when we are sleep deprived, we choose calorie-dense foods that are high in fat and sugar, and the metabolism slows down so that the body conserves as much energy as possible. This leads directly to weight gain, especially in the midsection.

In the long term, this is unsustainable and is a direct and important contributor to disease.

Common Sleep Thieves

- Taking the day's "unfinished business" and work problems to bed
- Going to bed angry, anxious, or afraid
- Heavy meals at night causing gas, indigestion, and acid reflux

- Alcohol, caffeine, and cigarettes
- Aches, pains, and illness
- Interruptions for urges to urinate
- An uncomfortable sleeping space with noise (such as snoring) or light
- Anxiety from the "first-night effect," or insomnia resulting from sleeping in an unfamiliar bed, such as in a hotel room

Improving Your Sleep Habits

The ultimate goal with our sleep habits is to get our biological clock in sync with nature. So arrange your bedroom window coverings so that natural light enters the room, especially in the morning hours. Then, spend at least part of each day outdoors, ideally with your bare feet touching the earth; this has an amazing effect on sleep.

Finally, develop a calming routine in the last hours before bedtime. Engage in relaxing and enjoyable endeavors, such as meditating, listening to calming music, or reading. Try to go to bed within a couple of hours of sunset; the most critical sleep time is from 10 PM to 2 AM.

Use the following tips to improve your sleep routine:

- Avoid alcohol, especially three to four hours before bedtime.
- Plan your fluid intake so that you are not waking up repeatedly to urinate.
- Dim your bedroom lights and limit your electronic screen time just before bedtime and in bed. The blue

light from your computer, phone, tablet, or TV screen is toxic to melatonin production.[7]

- Think "red before bed." Red-light lamps are calming (although red underwear might help with certain bedroom activities, which is good for sleep, too).
- Avoid caffeinated beverages six to eight hours before going to sleep.
- Do not eat heavy meals or exercise within three to four hours of bedtime.
- Avoid strenuous exercise in the evening, although a post-dinner stroll can really help.
- Physical factors like a firm mattress and pillows make a big difference.
- Keep your bedroom cool (around sixty-five to sixty-seven degrees) and pitch-dark. It's good for cuddling, too!
- Wear light and breathable night clothes, or better yet, try sleeping in the nude (also good for cuddling).
- Massage and intimate touch work wonders; sex is the best sleep aid!

CASE STUDY: MARGARET

Margaret, a forty-seven-year-old homemaker with three young children, was referred to me by her physician to help with weight control and type 2 diabetes. She was feeling like a "lost cause" because nothing she did seemed to work. She was tired, sleepless, constantly irritable, and generally unhappy with life.

Within a few weeks of starting my program, she felt her "old self" returning. She started to make sleep and stress reduction a priority. Simultaneously, the weight and fat that she had put on with three pregnancies started coming off, almost effortlessly. In two months, she had lost nine pounds and three inches off her waist circumference. Her doctor was also delighted that her blood pressure had improved twenty points, and her HbA1c dropped from 8.9 percent, which correlates with an average blood sugar of 209, to 7 percent, which correlates with an average blood sugar of 154.

CASE STUDY: STEVE

Steve, a fifty-two-year-old sales professional, struggled for years with diabetes and weight gain. Always an active person, he awoke at 5 AM to work out almost every day. With a stressful job, however, he would drink many cups of coffee and eat mindlessly to help cope with the stress and fatigue.

Committing to my program was transformative for Steve. It helped him realize that sleep deprivation was behind a lot of his cravings for sugary, fatty, and salty foods, and the large quantity of caffeine was leaving him "wired and tired."

Since starting the program, Steve has been getting seven to eight hours of quality sleep and has lost eleven pounds. He dropped two inches from his waist in two months, while decreasing his blood pressure twenty points. His HbA1c dropped from 8.6 percent, which correlates with an average blood sugar of 200, to 7.4 percent, which correlates with a blood sugar level of 166.

RULES TO LIVE BY

- Sleep is the most neglected master lever of health.
- Most of us are not getting enough quality sleep.
- Sleep directly affects appetite, food choice, and cravings.
- Sleep is one of the most important determinants of your immune system health.
- Sleep affects brain health: memory, mood, and pain perception.
- Make the conditions for quality sleep a priority during your waking hours.
- We need bedtime relaxation routines just like our children do.

CHAPTER NINE

Battling Environmental Enemies

Some days he walked along the banks of the river that smelled of shit
and pesticides bought with World Bank loans.
— ARUNDHATI ROY, *The God of Small Things*

Our increasingly synthetic world is immersed in unnatural chemicals. Many of these chemicals are ubiquitous environmental substances — toxins known to disrupt the normal functioning of the body's natural systems. These toxins interfere with your quest to attain Turbo Metabolism. Did you know that we are exposed to over a hundred harmful chemicals every morning even before we leave the house?[1]

Women are exposed to more harmful chemicals than men because they use more personal-care products, such as perfumes and cosmetics, though anyone in close proximity to these products is also affected.

Environmental toxins are often endocrine disruptors; that is, they can block hormones or actually impair the production of hormones by the endocrine glands. In other cases, they are toxic to our "inner garden" of a hundred trillion gut bacteria, which are trying to help us by busily producing beneficial substances. Many toxins are poisonous for mitochondria, the energy-producing component of every cell and our best friends in the quest for Turbo Metabolism (see chapter 6). In other words, these chemicals literally sap energy, short-circuit our power supply, and leave us tired, hungry, fat, and sick.

Environmental Toxins, Pollutants, and Preservatives

Here are a few of the main culprits of the 140 or so environmental pollutants to which most of us are exposed every day. They gain access to our bodies through food, water, our skin, and even the air we breathe.

The good news is that many of them (such as BPA, phthalates, and parabens) are not *persistent*, meaning that if we can minimize our daily exposure, they will leave our bodies quickly. However, some, like persistent organic pollutants and dioxins, can linger in the body for a long time.

Bisphenol A (BPA): Bisphenol A (BPA) has been linked to breast cancer, obesity, early puberty, and heart disease. About 93 percent of Americans have BPA in their bodies.[2] BPA sources include plastics, canned goods, and heat-sensitive paper (used in gas station, grocery store, and restaurant receipts). BPA is also found in meat packaging. The good news? If you can avoid exposure to BPA, levels in the body drop rapidly.

Phthalates: Plasticizers used to make plastics more soft and flexible, phthalates are commonly found in toys, hoses, toothbrushes, food packaging, shower curtains, synthetic fragrances (including most perfumes, and labeled as "added fragrance"), shampoos, hair spray, plastic spoons, and plastic wrap made from PVC with recycling label 3. They can trigger cell death in testicular cells, leading to lower sperm counts, less mobile sperm, and birth defects.[3] In addition to affecting the male reproductive system, they contribute to obesity, diabetes, and thyroid irregularities.[4] It is ironic that we use perfumes to attract people to us, but they actually impair our sexual performance. The good news is that they are nonpersistent. They can wash out of the body relatively quickly when we discontinue exposure.

Parabens: Parabens are commonly used as preservatives in skin products, such as shampoos, lotions, and creams (including many expensive "antiaging skin products"). They are also found in food, such as store-bought cinnamon rolls and cakes. An estrogen (female hormone) mimic, it has long been known for disrupting hormone function in animals.[5] Researchers from the University of California at Berkeley have linked parabens to breast cancer.[6] The good news is that these chemicals do not persist in the body; the bad news is that we re-expose ourselves every day.

Dioxins: Dioxins form during many industrial processes when chlorine or bromine are burned in the presence of carbon and oxygen. Dioxins interfere with both male and female reproductive function. Exposure in women early in life may permanently affect fertility.[7] In men, sperm quality and sperm count may be affected, causing infertility.[8] Dioxins are very long-lived and build up within the body and the food chain; in general, all toxins tend to become more prevalent as we move up the food chain. Dioxins are powerful carcinogens, and they may affect the immune system.[9] Dioxins are mainly found in products containing meat, fish, milk, and eggs. You can cut down your exposure to dioxins by eating fewer animal products, which means eating a plant-based diet.

Persistent organic pollutants (POPs): Persistent organic pollutants (POPs) include polychlorinated biphenyls (PCBs), atrazine, and organotins. PCBs are the most commonly used pesticides in commercial agriculture. The way most synthetic pesticides work is by harming the ability of living things to reproduce or by harming their nervous systems. PCBs are mainly found in soil and sediment and in fatty parts of fish, meat, and dairy products. Fish and shellfish usually contain the highest PCB levels of any food, especially fish that are fatty, that eat many other fish, and that are caught near industrial areas.

Atrazine is widely used as an herbicide spray in corn crops in the United States, and it is commonly found in drinking water because it gets into groundwater. Researchers have found that a low level of atrazine can turn male frogs into females that produce completely viable eggs![10] Atrazine has been linked to breast tumors, delayed puberty, and prostate inflammation in animals.[11]

Organotins are organic and inorganic tin compounds, used as fungicides, as stabilizers in plastics, as molluscicides (to kill snails), and as miticides (to kill mites). They have also been used as insect killers and for other industrial uses. Many of these products are unpalatable when mixed into diets and have been used as rodent repellent. Food chain accumulation and bioconcentration have been demonstrated in crabs, oysters, and salmon exposed to POPs. Not-so-fun fact: DDT is an example of a POP that was banned after it was found to be behind the shrinking population of bald eagles.

Triclosan: Triclosan is a known endocrine disruptor that affects thyroid function as well as liver toxicity. It is commonly used in body washes, antibacterial soap, and antibacterial toothpaste. Though it is included in toothpaste to fight gum disease and bad breath and labeled as such, it also "carpet bombs" healthy gut bacteria, which influences food choices, appetite, and ultimately weight and metabolic diseases.

Perfluorinated chemicals (PFCs): Perfluorinated chemicals (PFCs) are used to make nonstick cookware, an invention designed to get us to use less oil in cooking during the low-fat mania. They are so persistent that 99 percent of Americans are estimated to have these chemicals in their bodies.[12] PFCs are clearly linked with reproductive health, kidney disease, thyroid disease, high cholesterol, and many other health issues.[13] Animal studies suggest that PFCs can affect thyroid and sex hormone levels.[14]

Medications: Ironically, common prescription medications for treating diabetes, high blood pressure, and other metabolic diseases actually slow down metabolism and can cause weight gain. For example, a five-day regimen of antibiotics can destroy 33 percent of friendly gut bacteria, which affects mood and food choices. We now know that having a higher count of *Firmicutes* bacteria than *Bacteroidetes* bacteria in the gut microbiome is associated with weight gain.[15] This evidence is consistent with "feedlot efficiency" — the practice of giving antibiotics to feedlot cattle to increase weight gain by up to 30 percent.

Plastic contaminants: The familiar "chasing arrows" symbol on plastic containers and other plastic products does not mean the product is recyclable. The little number inside the triangle tells the real story. Within each chasing arrows triangle is a number ranging from 1 to 7. The purpose of the number is to identify the type of plastic used for the product, and not all plastics are recyclable or even reusable. Numerous plastic-based products cannot be recycled.

Products with recycling number 7 are the worst (think: unlucky 7). The number 7 category was designed as a catchall for polycarbonate (PC) and "other" plastics, so reuse and recycling protocols are not standardized within this category. Of primary concern with number 7 plastics, however, is the potential for chemical leaching into food or drink products packaged in polycarbonate containers made using BPA (see above). BPA is a xeno-estrogen (*xeno* means "foreign" or "other"), which is a known endocrine disruptor. Plastics with recycling numbers 2, 4, and 5 are better.

Arsenic: This poison lurks in your food and drinking water. If you ingest enough of it, arsenic will kill you outright. In smaller amounts, arsenic can cause skin, bladder, and lung cancer.[16] It is less well known that arsenic messes with your hormones! Specifically, it can interfere with normal hormone functioning in the glucocorticoid system that regulates how our bodies process sugars and carbohydrates.

Environmental Working Group Produce Recommendations

The Environmental Working Group (EWG) is an excellent nonprofit, nonpartisan organization dedicated to protecting human health and the environment. The mission of the EWG is to empower people to live healthier lives in a healthier environment. Publishing breakthrough research and providing educational resources, the organization drives consumer choice and civic action.

On its website, EWG publishes a ranking of common produce based on pesticide load. This ranking, as well as a database of potentially harmful household and personal-care products and other practical information, is available at EWG.org.

One thing I learned on this website is that washing and peeling nonorganic, store-bought produce does not solve the problem because the pesticide is sprayed into the soil and absorbed into the plant.

The USDA does not strictly define or regulate the use of the word "natural" except in the meat category. This means a tub of "all-natural yogurt" could legally contain synthetic pesticides, GMOs (genetically modified organisms), antibiotics, and growth hormones. The label "organic," however, requires that toxic, persistent synthetic pesticides and herbicides are not allowed, and neither are GMOs, antibiotics, growth hormones, or irradiation.

The EWG has done a good job of listing produce in order of pesticide load (highest to lowest). Because buying everything organic can be cost-prohibitive, being aware of which items of produce are highest in pesticide load is very helpful. In the list below, buying organic forms of only the first twelve items (the "dirty dozen") can reduce your pesticide exposure by up to 80 percent.[17] For a grower to certify and sell produce as "organic," the grower must undergo seven consecutive years of soil-testing for synthetic pesticides, herbicides, and petroleum-based (and sewage sludge–based) fertilizers. Also, organic certified crops cannot be genetically modified or irradiated. Genetic modification is often used to make corn and soy more pesticide tolerant (the crop lives but all the insects and weeds get killed), allowing it to be sprayed abundantly with these harmful chemicals. When these pesticides and herbicides (like Roundup) enter the body, they wreak havoc on the delicate ecosystem of gut bacteria.

The way these synthetic pesticides and herbicides are designed to work is by disrupting the endocrine (hormone) systems of the bugs or poisoning their nervous systems (neurotoxicity). This explains why we are seeing so much more infertility and neurodegenerative disorders in humans, such as Parkinson's disease, multiple sclerosis, and Alzheimer's, especially in farming communities.

What is the main problem with petroleum-based fertilizers? Using nitrogen-phosphorus-potassium (NPK) fertilizers creates shorter root systems, leading to lower micronutrient levels and compromised immunity to disease, requiring even higher levels of intervention. Using synthetic fertilizers, which are common in modern agriculture, is like providing a "junk food diet" to crops.

The 2017 EWG Ranking of Produce Based on Pesticide Load

Below is EWG's 2017 ranking of produce based on most to least exposure to pesticides, herbicides, and synthetic fertilizer. The top twelve are called the "dirty dozen"; buy these organic whenever possible.

EWG consistently ranks apples among the worst in terms of pesticide load. The average age of an apple in the grocery store is between four and eleven months, which may be why the soil around apple trees has to be so heavily saturated with pesticides.[18] The industry term "birthday apples" is sometimes used because apples sold in supermarkets are often one year old! Washing and peeling does not help because the harmful chemicals are inside the fruit.

1. Strawberries
   (the worst)
2. Spinach
3. Nectarines
4. Apples
5. Peaches
6. Pears
7. Cherries
8. Grapes
9. Celery
10. Tomatoes
11. Sweet bell peppers
12. Potatoes
13. Cucumbers
14. Cherry tomatoes
15. Lettuce
16. Snap peas (imported)
17. Blueberries
    (domestic)
18. Hot peppers
19. Kale / collard greens
20. Blueberries
    (imported)
21. Green beans
    (domestic)
22. Plums
23. Tangerines
24. Raspberries
25. Carrots
26. Winter squash
27. Oranges
28. Summer squash
29. Green beans
    (imported)
30. Snap peas (domestic)
31. Bananas
32. Green onions
33. Watermelon
34. Mushrooms
35. Sweet potatoes
36. Broccoli
37. Grapefruit
38. Cauliflower
39. Cantaloupe
40. Kiwi
41. Honeydew melon
42. Eggplant
43. Mangoes
44. Asparagus
45. Papayas
46. Sweet peas (frozen)
47. Onions
48. Cabbage
49. Pineapples
50. Avocados
51. Sweet corn

CASE STUDY: ANDREW

Andrew, a sixty-seven-year-old retired business owner, underwent a quadruple bypass operation nine years ago. When he became my patient, he started eating "clean and green," removing harmful chemicals and pesticides from his diet and choosing personal products that did not contain toxicants. He started to get lean and reclaim his energy, youth, and vitality that his old lifestyle and surgery had stolen from him.

Andrew now walks ten thousand steps every day, eats plant-based foods, meditates every day, and sleeps like a baby. His new mission in life is to spread the message of health and wellness to everyone he meets.

RULES TO LIVE BY

- Environmental pollutants and toxins are everywhere, so avoidance is key.
- When you enter your home, take off your shoes so that you do not bring in unwanted chemicals. Change into dedicated indoor shoes or sandals.
- Decrease or eliminate animal fats.
- Check your public water source (see chapter 5).
- If your tap water is sub-optimal, use a water filtration system (I prefer reverse osmosis systems) or drink filtered spring water.
- Wash your hands before you eat (but avoid harsh antibacterial soaps with chemicals like triclosan).
- Avoid plastic utensils and Styrofoam plates, especially when heating food (contaminants are released when

these are heated). Stainless steel or even bamboo are much better.

- Throw away scratched nonstick pans, which release PFCs. Stainless-steel pans are probably the best.
- Avoid printed receipts (most printers in commercial establishments use heat-sensitive paper loaded with BPA). Get electronic receipts, if possible.
- Insist on environmentally friendly dry-cleaning chemicals.
- Buy organic produce when possible.

CHAPTER TEN

Superfoods and Supplements

To grow the plants and animals that made up my meal, no pesti-cides found their way into any farmworker's bloodstream, no nitro-gen runoff or growth hormones seeped into the watershed, no soils were poisoned, no antibiotics were squandered, no subsidy checks were written. If the high price of my all-organic meal is weighed against the comparatively low price it exacted from the larger world, as it should be, it begins to look, at least in karmic terms, like a real bargain.

— MICHAEL POLLAN

The mind is everything. What you think, you become.

— BUDDHA

Is there such a thing as a superfood, or is there only food and nonfood? If a food makes you feel great not only while you are eating but also hours after you are done, this is probably a superfood for you. But as we scour the latest research, it turns out that there are some superfoods that cleanse, detoxify, and heal the body.

In reality, food is so much more than calories, fat, carbohydrates, protein, vitamins, and minerals. It is the most intimate and profound way in which we interact with the universe. The energy and intelligence of our food is far more important than the biochemical components that we tend to reduce it to.

What we eat can quite literally turn on or off our health and vitality. Only 2 percent of our genes actually code for the production of protein messengers; the other 98 percent simply send signals, determining which of the 2 percent of coding genes actually turn on. Quite literally, this means that environmental influences are a lot more powerful than our predetermined genetic code for health or disease.

The food we eat and the signals it provides determine our moods, our cravings, and our appetite as well as the vitamin production and vitality of our immune system. They determine how well we are able to cleanse, nourish, and detoxify our entire system, the inner garden.

Eating the right food requires mindful attention. It requires knowing what we are hungry for and distinguishing between nutritional deficiencies, thirst, emotional hunger, need for variety, low blood sugar, and a true "empty stomach" hunger. Eating right is about giving the body what it needs to help us feel nourished and energized. It means eating fresh, wholesome, in-season local food, and avoiding the food felons of sugar, corn syrup, refined grains, and trans and saturated fats. It means eating mostly fresh vegetables and fruit, very high fiber, and lots of omega-3 fats. It means getting the full range of plant nutrients by putting all the colors of the rainbow on your plate. It means keeping the glycemic load low and sodium intake low while minimizing consumption of animal products (especially dairy) to maintain ideal hormone balance.

The best superfood for human consumption may be human

breast milk. Because infants lack the enzymes to digest *oligo-saccharides* in human breast milk, these oligosaccharides nourish *Bifidobacterium infantis*, which keeps the infant healthy by nurturing the lining of the intestines and protecting the infant from infection and inflammation. Human breast milk is the perfect *pre*biotic (meaning food for the healthy bacteria in the gut) and *pro*biotic (meaning the actual health-promoting gut bacteria themselves). Breast milk is prebiotic because it contains oligosaccharides: food for the healthy bacteria. It is probiotic because it promotes a healthy gut microbiome.

But if you're reading this book, there's a good chance that you're not drinking breast milk any longer.

Facts and Fallacies

- Your gut bacteria influence your weight.

  ⅠⅠⅠⅡ➡ Fact

  Gut bacterial composition can influence hunger cravings and weight gain. This is disturbed by synthetic chemicals, such as antibiotics added to animal feed and also artificial sweeteners.

- The most searched vitamin on the internet is vitamin C.

  ⅠⅠⅠⅡ➡ Fact

  Since the Nobel Prize–winning work of Linus Pauling, many more benefits of vitamin C have been discovered. Citrus fruits, like limes and lemons (which I recommend eating every day), are rich in vitamin C.

Good Bacteria, Superfoods, and Turbo Metabolism

The typical human adult has far more bacterial cells than human cells in their body; in fact, we have about ten times as much bacterial DNA as human DNA!

These bacteria protect us by helping to produce vitamins, detoxify harmful substances that we ingest, break down fat, and regulate cholesterol. There is a gut-brain connection, and our moods, concentration, attention, and even our food preferences and cravings might be a result of the kind of bacteria that reside in our gut (for instance, by producing serotonin and melatonin; see chapter 8).

So what can you do to have a healthy gastrointestinal microbiome? The gastrointestinal system (or "gut") includes all the digestive organs from the mouth to the anus — the largest numbers of good bacteria reside in the large intestine or colon.

Superfoods help optimize that symbiotic/collaborative relationship between these microorganisms and our bodies and move us toward Turbo Metabolism. When we have the right types of healthy bacteria in the right quantities and ratios, they can profoundly affect our food choices, our appetite, our immune system — and even brain function — to help move the body toward a state of optimal balance. This is the goal of Turbo Metabolism.

The scientific evidence suggests that a nutrient-dense, plant-rich diet of unprocessed food, a diet that's high in both soluble and insoluble fiber, as well as resistant starch, can increase the population of a healthy gut microbiome. A diet rich in these superfoods will help nourish you while detoxifying and cleansing your system, decreasing inflammation, and promoting healthy hormonal balance.[1]

Cruciferous vegetables: Examples of cruciferous vegetables are cauliflower, broccoli, Brussels sprouts, and cabbage. Broccoli sprouts especially reduce oxidative stress, inflammation, insulin resistance, and fasting blood sugars. Broccoli contains *sulforaphane*, which is released about forty minutes after cutting the sprouts. These sulfur-containing vegetables actually detoxify the body of metabolic poisons and kill precancerous cells before they turn into cancer.

High-nutrient vegetables: Kale, collard greens, and spinach are good examples of high-nutrient vegetables. These vegetables are rich in anti-inflammatory and oxidative flavonoids and carotenoids: vitamins A, B_2, B_6, C, E, and K, along with calcium, folate, potassium, magnesium, iron, manganese, and tryptophan. They also contain *glucosinolates*, which have cancer-preventative benefits.[2]

Legumes: Legumes include all types of beans (such as red, black, brown, yellow, and navy beans), in addition to lentils, peas, and especially chickpeas. Legumes provide the prebiotic-resistant starch needed by healthy gut bacteria. As a by-product of their metabolism by good bacteria, legumes contain short-chain fatty acids such as *butyrate*, which is known to improve insulin sensitivity, protect from colon cancer, and help absorb minerals, such as magnesium and calcium.[3] Butyrate also has several anti-inflammatory activities.[4] Legumes are also an excellent source of fiber, both soluble and insoluble.

However, if you are diabetic with significant carbohydrate sensitivity, beans and legumes might spike your blood glucose. Frequent blood-glucose testing (both before and one to two hours after eating) is the only way to find out if that is the case with you.

Mushrooms: Mushrooms, especially shiitake and maitake, promote *immune globulin A*, which is crucial for defending the mucous membrane — the delicate lining in the nose and mouth that extends throughout the respiratory and gastrointestinal passages. This lining maintains a barrier against harmful invaders. Mushrooms have also been shown to boost the immune system.[5]

Grains: Unprocessed whole-kernel grains (not flour), such as barley, black wild rice, and oats, are low-glycemic, meaning they generally do not spike blood-sugar levels. These grains are loaded with resistant starch, as well as soluble and insoluble fiber, which act as prebiotic food for healthy gut bacteria. These grains are also a good source of plant protein. If you are diabetic, you still need to be careful and monitor your own blood-sugar response to come up with your own eating plan.

Nuts: Nuts, especially almonds and walnuts, are rich in healthy fats and help improve arterial function while lowering cholesterol oxidation. Nut consumption has been directly correlated with reduction in sudden cardiac death (death from heart rhythm irregularity in the absence of preceding heart disease).[6] However, you should be careful how many nuts you eat because they can be calorie dense; a handful a day is enough. Eating a handful of almonds or walnuts thirty minutes before eating your regular meal can help promote satiety and suppress appetite quite a bit.

Avocados: Avocados are a great source of complex carbohydrates and healthy fat, which creates satiety and nourishes the mitochondria.

Sweet potatoes: Sweet potato is a relatively low-glycemic food with protein (all the essential amino acids) and some fat as well. It's also a good source of lysine, making it a nice complement to grains.

Other prebiotic foods: Prebiotic foods promote healthy bacteria in the gut. You should keep in mind that eating probiotics either from supplements or from food sources (such as yogurt, sauerkraut, or kimchee) — without accompanying them with prebiotic foods — is really only a Band-Aid solution. Probiotic bacteria survive only a few hours to a few days; they need to have prebiotic food to be able to reproduce before they die. Here are some examples of the best prebiotic foods:

- Apples
- Asparagus
- Bananas
- Chicory root
- Garlic
- Jerusalem artichokes
- Kiwi
- Onions, leeks
- Peas

Detoxifying foods: Detoxifying foods help digestion and excretion by capturing harmful chemicals and pushing them out of the body through the urine or feces. Here are some good detoxifying foods:

- Beets
- Berries
- Cruciferous vegetables
- Garlic
- Green tea
- Okra
- Onions

Anti-inflammatory Spices

Spices have been used for thousands of years to enhance flavor and also to help us absorb and metabolize nutrients optimally. It could be argued that the search for spices was behind the discovery of the New World by European explorers.

Turmeric: Studies have shown that turmeric reduces insulin resistance in both prediabetes and type 2 diabetes. It also has significant anti-inflammatory properties (as measured by tumor necrosis factor, or TNF, expression).[7] Currently, curcumin, which is the active ingredient in turmeric, is a hot research topic in the world of cancer prevention and treatment as well.

Rosemary: Rosemary protects brain cells from oxidative damage, reducing the risk of Parkinson's disease and Alzheimer's disease.[8] It also decreases the production of carcinogenic chemicals from charred meats if added to marinade.[9]

Ginger: In addition to having potent anti-inflammatory effects, ginger is also very good for alleviating nausea and improving gut health.[10] Traditionally used to promote digestive health for many millennia, it helps with acid reflux and flatulence.

Cloves: Cloves and their oil have been used medicinally for pain relief for millennia. They have significant anti-inflammatory properties, as measured by tumor necrosis factor (TNF) expression.[11]

Mustard seeds: Mustard seeds help with digestion and release beneficial compounds such as sulforaphanes from cruciferous vegetables like broccoli.[12]

Black pepper: In addition to enhancing flavor and promoting digestion and intestinal motility, black pepper helps release beneficial curcumin from turmeric.[13]

Cinnamon: In addition to being a great substitute for sugar, cinnamon benefits diabetics by reducing fasting blood glucose by 18 to 29 percent in some studies.[14]

Vitamin and Mineral Supplements

As the term implies, the idea is to use vitamins and minerals to *supplement* your optimal nutrition, exercise, stress management, and sleep strategies, from which you will derive 90 percent of your health benefits. Readers and patients often make the mistake of thinking that supplements are the silver bullet that will "neutralize" important core factors. This is not true. Correct supplementation will give you a slight edge, but the main emphasis should be on the food you eat: focus on a nutrient-dense, plant-rich diet.

Ideally, supplementation should be based on individual needs, but some generalizations can be made. My suggestion is to first think about optimizing omega-3 oils, vitamin D, and magnesium. After those, consider the other supplements, as there is some evidence that they offer additional benefit over and above optimal food choices. But again, you will get the most bang for your buck by eating the right foods, while supplements can give you perhaps a 10 percent additional benefit.

Vitamin D: Vitamin D is made from cholesterol in the skin in response to UV light. Up to 70 percent of Americans have vitamin D deficiency.[15] Because there are no good dietary sources of vitamin D and we spend most of our time indoors, vitamin D is an important supplement. The liver converts vitamin D to 25-hydroxy vitamin D, which acts as a hormone in the body.

Vitamin D is involved in hundreds of enzymatic (chemical) reactions in the body and is known to affect various metabolic

parameters, such as HDL (good) cholesterol. HDL cholesterol increases in direct correlation with 25-hydroxy vitamin D.
Vitamin D is important for weight and metabolism, immune
modulation, and pain. Low vitamin D is strongly associated
with depression and also autism.[16] Optimization of vitamin
D level correlates with reduction in risk of death from breast,
colon, and prostate cancer.[17]

I recommend 2,000 international units (IU) of vitamin D
daily.

Omega-3 oils: Omega-3 oils come from cold-water marine life
such as fish or algae. They are vitally important for maintaining arterial lining and cell membranes and for heart and brain
health in general.[18] These oils help maintain healthy fats in the
bloodstream and improve HDL cholesterol levels.[19] Research
indicates that they may also be very important for mental health
and memory.[20]

I recommend 500 mg of both EPA (eicosapentaenoic acid)
and DHA (docosahexaenoic acid) omega-3 oils daily. Ideally,
you can get this from plant sources (algae derived), but a high-
quality fish oil would also suffice.

Magnesium: Magnesium helps the coordination between the
nerves and muscles; it is also involved in hundreds of enzymatic
processes in the body. It aids with improving insulin sensitivity, blood-pressure control, and circulation, as well as sleep. Up
to 40 percent of Americans have a magnesium deficiency because of a lack of green leafy vegetables in the typical US diet.[21]
Greens are the best source, as magnesium is at the center of
the chlorophyll molecule. This means eating a nutrient-dense,
plant-rich diet is the best way to get magnesium.

As a supplement, I recommend 400 mg of magnesium daily.

Coenzyme Q10: Levels of coenzyme Q10 (CoQ10) are depleted in the body as we get older; this occurs especially when certain medications, such as statins, are taken regularly.[22] Coenzyme Q10 is vital for heart health and healthy circulation.

I recommend 100 mg of CoQ10 daily.

Alpha lipoic acid: Alpha lipoic acid (ALA) has been shown to be beneficial for diabetes control (especially for diabetes neuropathy) by promoting mitochondrial health.

I recommend from 1,200 to 1,800 mg of alpha lipoic acid daily.

Vitamin B$_{12}$: Vitamin B$_{12}$ can be especially important for those following a strict vegan eating plan because vitamin B$_{12}$ is made by microorganisms. Therefore, it would be lacking in a strict vegan diet.

For those people, I recommend 1,000 mcg of vitamin B$_{12}$ daily.

Other supplements: You may gain some additional benefit from chromium picolinate, which has been shown to improve insulin sensitivity because it acts as an insulin cofactor.[23] Also, studies show that apple cider vinegar slows down the release of sugar into the bloodstream after a starchy meal.[24] Take a half teaspoon of apple cider vinegar before meals (perhaps dissolved in water) or in salad dressing.

RULES TO LIVE BY

- Focus on changing your *core* lifestyle factors — diet/nutrition, stress reduction, sleep habits, and social support. Supplement intake is a *satellite* measure.

- Superfoods for turbocharging your metabolism are beans, cruciferous vegetables, leafy greens, nuts, and seeds.
- Targeted (individualized) vitamin/mineral therapy can help.
- Vitamin D, fish oil, magnesium, alpha lipoic acid, and vitamin B_{12} are the most important supplements.

CHAPTER ELEVEN

Turbo Metabolism Recipes

To feed oneself wholesomely is the most profound and powerful way to achieve good health. I have collected these quick and easy recipes over the years with the intention of creating tasty, healthy meals. The goal is to nourish and nurture the body with simple ingredients and to get more whole-plant foods into your diet. Always remember that my program is not just a diet; it's a lifestyle geared to eliminating foods and behaviors that make you weak and tired and replacing them with foods and behaviors that make you stronger.

With that in mind, here are my favorite breakfast, Indian, Asian, Southwestern, Mexican, pasta, and veggie side dishes, plus salads, soups, and snack options. All the Indian recipes are from my mom's kitchen as they have been passed down for centuries. Many others are courtesy of a few like-minded colleagues and friends: Joel Fuhrman, MD, from his *Eat to Live Cookbook*; Dr. Cathi Misquitta and Dr. Rajiv Misquitta, from their *Healthy Heart, Healthy Planet* cookbook; and Joel Kahn, MD, author of *The Plant-Based Solution* and other books.

Whenever possible, purchase certified organic ingredients,

ideally ones that are locally grown. And don't worry too much about adhering rigidly to the ingredient lists and instructions — start with what you have, and if you put some love into it, the result will always be delightful. I hope you'll have fun preparing these dishes — and find that turbocharging your metabolism is satisfying and delicious!

Breakfast

Snacks

Salads and Soups

Indian and Asian

Southwestern and Mexican

Pasta

Veggie Sides

BREAKFAST

Turbo Metabolism Breakfast Bowl

This quick breakfast fix is loaded with fiber, healthy fats, and antioxidants. Mulberries are a superfood with blood sugar–regulating properties and the potent antioxidant resveratrol. They look like tiny golden pinecones and are available dried in natural-food stores or online.

Makes 1 serving

¼ cup high-fiber oat bran
2 tablespoons chia seeds
2 tablespoons hemp seeds
¼ cup raisins
¼ cup mulberries
½ cup blueberries
1 tablespoon almond butter
1 cup boiling water

In a serving bowl, combine the oat bran, chia seeds, hemp seeds, raisins, mulberries, blueberries, and almond butter. Add the boiling water, and mix with a spoon until the oat bran appears moist and takes on a semisolid consistency.

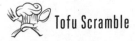 ## Tofu Scramble

Recipe adapted from Healthy Heart, Healthy Planet *by Dr. Cathi Misquitta and Dr. Rajiv Misquitta*

Since the Turbo Metabolism diet favors plant-based foods over animal proteins, I recommend eating scrambled tofu on the weekends instead of eggs when you want a savory brunch. This recipe is packed with nutrients and flavor.

1 onion, diced
⅔ cup seeded and chopped shishito or green bell peppers
1 cup diced shimeji (oyster) or button mushrooms
1 package (16 ounces) organic firm tofu, drained and crumbled
½ teaspoon curry powder
Dash of ground turmeric
1 cup fresh spinach
1 tomato, diced
Salt
Pepper
1 slice whole-grain toast (optional)
Hummus (optional)

In a dry, nonstick skillet over medium heat, sauté the onion, peppers, and mushrooms until the onion turns translucent, about 5 to 7 minutes. Stir in the tofu, curry powder, and turmeric, and cook for 2 minutes, or until the tofu is warmed through. Reduce the heat to low, add the spinach and tomato, and cook for about 2 more minutes, or until the spinach is wilted. Season with salt and pepper to taste. Serve with toast and hummus, if desired, to complete the brunch.

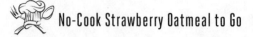 No-Cook Strawberry Oatmeal to Go

Recipe adapted from Eat to Live Cookbook *by Joel Fuhrman, MD*

Prepare this dish the night before so it's ready to go in the morning. Note that other berries, cherries, or sliced peaches may also be used instead of strawberries.

Makes 1 serving

⅓ cup old-fashioned rolled oats
1 tablespoon chia seeds
⅔ cup unsweetened soy, hemp, or almond milk
1 cup sliced fresh or thawed frozen strawberries
6 walnut halves, crushed

In a portable cup or bowl, combine the oats, chia seeds, and nondairy milk, and stir. Cover and refrigerate overnight. In the morning, stir in the strawberries and walnuts.

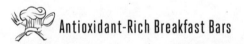 Antioxidant-Rich Breakfast Bars

Recipe adapted from Eat to Live Cookbook *by Joel Fuhrman, MD*

As the name implies, these bars are packed with diabesity-fighting antioxidants. They're also a great option for a quick, portable breakfast when you're in a hurry.

Makes 6 bars

1 medium ripe banana

1 cup old-fashioned oats

1 cup fresh or thawed frozen blueberries

¼ cup raisins

⅛ cup pomegranate juice

2 tablespoons finely chopped dates

1 tablespoon chopped walnuts

1 tablespoon goji berries or other unsulfured dried fruit

1 tablespoon raw sunflower seeds

2 tablespoons ground flaxseed

Olive oil

Preheat the oven to 350°F. In a large bowl, mash the banana. Add the oats, blueberries, raisins, pomegranate juice, dates, walnuts, goji berries, sunflower seeds, and flaxseed, and mix thoroughly.

Lightly wipe an 8-inch-square baking pan with a small amount of olive oil. Spread the mixture into the pan, and bake for 25 minutes. Cool on a wire rack, and then cut into bars. Store any remaining bars in the fridge for up to a week.

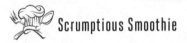 ## Scrumptious Smoothie

You can never go wrong with a tasty smoothie for breakfast. In this one, the ginger and lemon help digestion. Use more or fewer greens depending on the type of green and your tolerance for the flavor — experiment!

1–2 handfuls organic greens (such as spinach, kale,
    or arugula)

ı organic apple, core removed
ı organic pear, core removed
½-inch piece fresh ginger
ı teaspoon almond butter
½ lemon, peeled
A few ice cubes or approximately ½ cup crushed ice

Place all ingredients in a high-powered blender, and blend until smooth.

SNACKS

Simple Whole-Food Snack Options

Periodic healthy snacking can help maintain stable blood glucose levels and prevent spikes and sharp drops in these levels. Here are a few ideas for simple go-to snacks.

- Raw almonds (6) or walnuts (10 halves)
- Fruits (such as berries, tangerine, orange, pear)
- Low-carb protein shake with unsweetened almond milk or soy milk, berries, and vegan protein powder made with pea or rice protein
- Half of an avocado

Guacamole with Celery Sticks

This fantastic Mexican dip is simple to make and delivers lots of healthy fat as well as the powerful antioxidant lycopene from the tomatoes and the digestive benefits of cayenne pepper.

2 avocados, halved and pitted
Juice of 1 lime
Pinch of salt
½ medium red onion, chopped
1 bunch cilantro, chopped
2 medium tomatoes, chopped
2 cloves garlic, minced
Pinch of cayenne pepper
Celery sticks

In a medium bowl, mash the avocados. Stir in the lime juice, salt, onion, cilantro, tomatoes, garlic, and cayenne. Refrigerate for 1 hour for best flavor, or serve immediately. Eat with celery sticks.

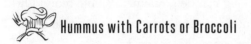 ## Hummus with Carrots or Broccoli

Hummus — a healthy Mediterranean dip that makes anything taste better! Enjoy with some vegetables for a delightful superfood snack.

1 cup drained cooked chickpeas (canned is fine)
2 cloves garlic
½ teaspoon olive oil
½ teaspoon tahini
Dash of fresh lemon juice

Blend all ingredients in a blender until smooth. Store any unused hummus in a sealed container in the fridge for up to a week.

SALADS AND SOUPS

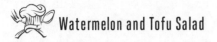 ### Watermelon and Tofu Salad

Recipe adapted from Healthy Heart, Healthy Planet *by Dr. Cathi Misquitta and Dr. Rajiv Misquitta*

This cooling summer salad is a symphony of textures and flavors. Feel free to use white, red, or yellow miso paste — any of the three will work fine.

Makes 4 servings

1 package (16 ounces) organic firm tofu, drained and cut into
     ½-inch cubes
4 cups seeded cubed watermelon (1-inch cubes)
1 medium tomato, diced
¼ cup finely chopped parsley
¼ cup finely chopped mint
1 tablespoon miso
1 tablespoon lemon juice
1 tablespoon red wine vinegar

Preheat the oven to 450°F. Line a baking sheet with parchment paper. Place the tofu on the baking sheet and bake for 25 minutes. Let the tofu cool completely.

Transfer the tofu to a large bowl, add the watermelon, tomato, parsley, mint, miso, lemon juice, and vinegar, and mix well. Serve immediately.

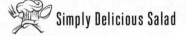 Simply Delicious Salad

For the greens in this salad, feel free to use mesclun mix, spinach, arugula, baby kale, or plain-old lettuce — whatever suits your fancy. You can also use whatever beans you like; chickpeas and black beans are my go-to varieties.

Makes 1 serving

2 cups salad greens
½ cup cooked beans (canned is fine)
1 rib celery, thinly sliced
1 fistful grape or cherry tomatoes
½ cup sliced mushrooms
1 tablespoon slivered almonds
1 handful organic berries
1 tablespoon pomegranate arils (seeds)
1 teaspoon fresh lime juice or 1 teaspoon Ginger Almond
    Dressing (recipe follows) (optional)

In a large bowl, toss together the greens, beans, celery, tomatoes, mushrooms, almonds, berries, and pomegranate arils. Drizzle with the fresh lime juice or Ginger Almond Dressing, if desired.

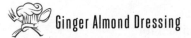 ## Ginger Almond Dressing

Recipe adapted from Eat to Live Cookbook *by Joel Fuhrman, MD*

This delicious nutty dressing is good on anything! It also works well as a veggie dip.

Makes approximately ¾ cup

¼ cup raw almond butter or ½ cup raw almonds
¼ cup unsweetened soy, hemp, or almond milk
¼ cup water
2 tablespoons rice vinegar
2 tablespoons unhulled sesame seeds
3 dates, pitted
2 small cloves garlic, coarsely chopped
½-inch piece fresh ginger, peeled and coarsely chopped

In a high-powered blender, blend all ingredients together until creamy. Add more water if a thinner dressing is desired.

Curried Rice Salad with Peppers and Raisins

Recipe adapted from Healthy Heart, Healthy Planet *by Dr. Cathi Misquitta and Dr. Rajiv Misquitta*

You'll love the zingy dressing on this crunchy, filling salad.

Makes 4 servings

Tofu-Curry Dressing
½ package (8 ounces) organic silken tofu
⅓ cup lemon juice
¼ cup rice vinegar
1 tablespoon curry powder

Rice and Vegetables
6 cups cooked wild rice
¾ cup raisins
3 stalks celery, diced
1 green bell pepper, diced
1 red bell pepper, diced
1 bunch green onions, diced
¼ red onion, diced
1 can (15 ounces) chickpeas, drained
Salt to taste

In a blender, combine the tofu, lemon juice, vinegar, and curry powder, and blend until smooth.

In a large bowl, mix the cooked rice, raisins, celery, green and red peppers, green and red onions, and chickpeas. Add salt to taste.

Pour the dressing over the rice and vegetables and mix well. Chill for 20 minutes and serve.

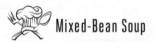 ## Mixed-Bean Soup

I like using ten-bean soup mix for this recipe, but you can make your own mixture — or even use all one kind of bean in a pinch.

Makes 4 servings

½ cup dried beans
½ teaspoon coconut oil or avocado oil
½ medium yellow onion, minced
1 clove garlic, chopped
1 rib celery, sliced
Pinch of salt
Pinch of pepper
Pinch of cumin seeds
Pinch of ground turmeric
2 cups water
2 medium tomatoes

In a medium bowl, cover the beans with 1 inch of water and leave them to soak for at least 8 hours. In a large skillet, heat the oil over medium heat. Add the onion, garlic, celery, salt, pepper, cumin seeds, and turmeric. Cook for 7 to 10 minutes, or until the onion starts to change color to a pinkish hue.

Drain the beans and place them in a large slow-cooker or a large pot. Add the 2 cups water to cover the beans. Stir in the onion mixture. Add the tomatoes. If using a slow cooker, cover and cook on 180°F for 8 hours or until the beans are tender; if cooking on the stovetop, cover and cook over medium to high heat for about 45 minutes, or until the beans are tender.

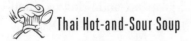 Thai Hot-and-Sour Soup

Recipe adapted from Healthy Heart, Healthy Planet *by Dr. Cathi Misquitta and Dr. Rajiv Misquitta*

Nothing beats the soothing flavors of a Thai curry. This soup calls for almond milk instead of the traditional coconut milk, resulting in a lighter soup with less saturated fat.

Makes 4 servings

4 cups low-sodium vegetable broth/stock or water
8 thin slices ginger
1 stalk lemongrass, cut into 1-inch-long pieces
1 tablespoon Thai red curry paste
3 tablespoons soy sauce
Zest and juice of 2 limes
2 cups unsweetened almond milk
2 tablespoons agave nectar
2 large shallots, thinly sliced
¼ cup Thai basil
½ jalapeño, seeded
1½ cups baby carrots
1 package (16 ounces) organic firm tofu, cubed
1 head bok choy, chopped
1 zucchini, cut in half lengthwise and then cut into
     ½-inch-wide semicircles
1½ cups halved cherry tomatoes
1 cup mung bean sprouts for garnish
Cilantro sprigs for garnish

In a large stockpot, combine the broth or water, ginger, lemon-grass, curry paste, soy sauce, lime zest and juice, almond milk, agave nectar, shallots, basil, and jalapeño, and bring to a boil. Add the carrots, turn the heat down to medium, and cook for 3 to 4 minutes. Add the tofu, bok choy, and zucchini, and cook for 3 to 4 more minutes. Add the tomatoes, and cook for an-other 2 to 3 minutes, or until the vegetables are tender. Serve in large bowls and garnish with bean sprouts and cilantro.

INDIAN AND ASIAN

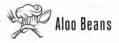 **Aloo Beans**

This recipe for potatoes and green beans is so easy, anyone can make it.

Makes 2 servings

2 tablespoons coconut oil or mustard oil
¼ teaspoon mustard seeds
½ teaspoon cumin seeds
2½ cups French beans, cut into ½-inch pieces
1 cup chopped potatoes
¼ teaspoon ground turmeric
½ teaspoon ground cumin
1 teaspoon ground coriander
1 teaspoon red chili powder
½ teaspoon garam masala
1 teaspoon lemon juice
Salt

In a large skillet over medium heat, heat the oil. Once hot, add the mustard seeds and let them pop. Then stir in the cumin seeds and let them sizzle. Stir in the beans, potatoes, turmeric, cumin, coriander, and chili powder. Cover the pan and cook covered, stirring occasionally, for 15 minutes, or until the vegetables are soft and tender. Stir in the garam masala, followed by the lemon juice. Add salt to taste. Serve immediately.

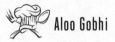 ## Aloo Gobhi

This side dish of cauliflower and potatoes is another super-easy, quick one.

Makes 4 servings

1 head cauliflower (approximately 1¾ pounds), cut into
     ¾-inch-wide florets
1¼ pounds Yukon Gold potatoes, peeled and cut into
     ½-inch cubes
5 tablespoons coconut oil or avocado oil, divided
½ teaspoon cumin seeds
¾ teaspoon salt, divided
1 medium onion, finely chopped
2 cloves garlic, finely chopped
2 teaspoons minced fresh jalapeño, including seeds
2 teaspoons minced peeled fresh ginger
1 teaspoon ground cumin
½ teaspoon ground coriander
¼ teaspoon ground turmeric
¼ teaspoon cayenne pepper
½ cup water
Lemon wedges for garnish (optional)

In a 12-inch skillet over medium heat, toss the cauliflower and potatoes with 3 tablespoons oil, the cumin seeds, and ¼ teaspoon salt. Cook, stirring occasionally, until the cauliflower is tender and browned in spots and the potatoes are just tender, about 20 minutes.

While the vegetables are cooking, in a separate 12-inch skillet over medium heat, cook the onion, garlic, jalapeño, and ginger in the remaining 2 tablespoons oil. Stirring frequently, cook until the vegetables are very soft and beginning to turn golden, 8 to 10 minutes. Add the cumin, coriander, turmeric, cayenne, and remaining ½ teaspoon salt and cook, stirring constantly, for 2 minutes more. Stir in the water, scraping up any brown bits from the bottom of the skillet, then stir in the cauliflower and potatoes. Cover and cook, stirring occasionally, for 5 more minutes. Serve immediately, with lemon wedges on the side, if desired.

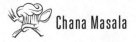 ## Chana Masala

Chana means "chickpeas," and *masala* means "spice."

Makes 4 servings

1 tablespoon olive oil
1 large onion, chopped
2–3 cloves garlic, minced
2 cans (30 ounces) chickpeas, drained and rinsed
1–2 teaspoons garam masala or good-quality curry powder
½ teaspoon ground turmeric
2 teaspoons grated fresh or jarred ginger
2 large tomatoes, diced
1 tablespoon lemon juice
¼ cup water
¼ cup minced fresh cilantro, or to taste
Salt

Hot cooked grain (rice, quinoa, or whole-wheat couscous)
   (optional)

In a large skillet, heat the oil over medium heat. Add the onion
and sauté until translucent, about 5 to 7 minutes. Add the garlic
and continue to sauté until the onion is golden, about 10 more
minutes.

Add the chickpeas, garam masala, turmeric, ginger, tomatoes, lemon juice, and water. Bring to a simmer, then cook,
uncovered, over medium-low heat for 10 minutes, stirring frequently. This should be moist and stew-like, but not soupy; add
a little more water, if needed.

Stir in the cilantro and season with salt to taste. Serve alone
in shallow bowls or over a hot cooked grain, if desired.

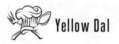 **Yellow Dal**

A dal is a pulse or legume, and it's also the name of the stews
that are made of these legumes. Dal can be eaten as a snack or
even a meal, especially if it's served over a bit of rice. Legumes
are high in fiber and protein and can be deliciously satisfying.

Makes 4 to 6 servings

Dal
1 cup split yellow lentils (moong dal)
3 cups water
½ teaspoon ground turmeric
Medium-grain kosher salt

Tarka (Seasoning)
2 tablespoons coconut oil
1 teaspoon cumin seeds
1 small onion, minced
1 or 2 fresh or dried whole red chilies

Leaves picked from a small bunch of cilantro
Fresh lime wedges for garnish

To make the dal, rinse the lentils. In a medium heavy saucepan, cover the lentils with water. Swish them around with your hand, then drain the water through a fine-mesh sieve. Return the lentils to the saucepan and repeat, washing, agitating, and draining, until the water runs absolutely clear. It will probably take seven to ten changes of water.

Once the lentils are clean, pour the 3 cups of water into the pot to cover them. Bring to a boil over medium-high heat, skim off any residue that rises to the surface, then lower the heat to maintain a simmer. Add the turmeric and cook until the dal is quite creamy, 45 to 60 minutes. Stir the lentils regularly as they simmer so that they don't catch at the bottom of the pan and burn. If the lentils start to look dry before they are cooked, add hot water (from the tap is fine). Season well with salt.

Start making the tarka about 20 minutes before the dal is done. In a pan, melt the coconut oil over low heat. Fry the cumin seeds for about 1 minute, until sizzling and fragrant. Add the onion and chilies and cook, stirring, until the onion is very soft and translucent, about 15 minutes. When the dal is ready, add the tarka to the dal, stirring to partially combine. Sprinkle the cilantro on top, and serve with lime wedges.

Bhindi

Bhindi is a dish of okra and onions. It's one of my kids' favorites: I can hear them say, "More bhindi, please." Note that okra can get sticky when cooked; to avoid this, cook uncovered and without salt. In properly cooked bhindi, the okra is slightly crisp and not mushy, with the seeds still inside.

Makes 4 servings

1 tablespoon avocado oil or coconut oil
1 green chili, finely chopped (I use serrano pepper).
1 medium onion, finely sliced
2 cups chopped fresh okra
¼ teaspoon ground turmeric
¾ teaspoon salt
Red chili powder (optional)

In a large skillet, heat the oil on medium. Add the green chili and cook for 2 minutes, stirring occasionally.

Add the onion and cook on medium-low heat until the onion starts to turn pink, about 6 to 8 minutes.

Add the okra and turmeric and cook uncovered on medium-low heat for 10 minutes. Stir only twice to prevent the okra from releasing its seeds. Once the okra is cooked to preference, remove from the stove. Add the salt and optional chili powder and gently mix. Serve hot.

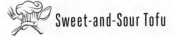 Sweet-and-Sour Tofu

Recipe adapted from Healthy Heart, Healthy Planet *by Dr. Cathi Misquitta and Dr. Rajiv Misquitta*

Yams are an excellent low-glycemic starch. They provide dietary fiber, B vitamins, and beta-carotene. And tangy pineapple makes the perfect complement in this flavor-packed dish.

Makes 6 servings

2 medium yams, scrubbed and cut into ¾-inch cubes
1 package (16 ounces) organic extra-firm tofu, cut into
    ¾-inch cubes
1 pineapple

Sweet-and-Sour Sauce
2 tomatoes, cut into 1-inch pieces
½-inch cube of fresh ginger
1 teaspoon garlic powder
3 tablespoons light soy sauce
⅓ cup lemon juice
⅓ cup rice vinegar
1 tablespoon cornstarch

Vegetables and Rice
2 carrots, peeled and sliced at an angle into ⅛-inch-thick
    pieces
1 yellow onion, cut into 1-inch pieces
1 green bell pepper, seeded and cut into 1-inch pieces
1 red bell pepper, seeded and cut into 1-inch pieces
6 cups cooked rice

Preheat the oven to 375°F. Line a baking sheet with parchment paper. Place the yams and tofu on the baking sheet and bake for 40 minutes.

To prepare the pineapple, slice off the top and bottom. Place the pineapple on its bottom edge, and slice downward from the top to remove the skin. "Eyes" may still need to be removed. If so, find a line of pineapple eyes, and slice along the outside edge of the eyes on either side. Continue until the pineapple is clean. Then, quarter the pineapple lengthwise. Place each quarter on its bottom edge, and slice downward to remove the pineapple core. Reserve half of the pineapple for the dish and half for the sauce. Cut each quarter lengthwise into 3 pieces, then cut crosswise into ¾-inch-wide pieces.

To make the sauce, in a blender, combine half of the pineapple and the tomatoes, ginger, garlic powder, soy sauce, lemon juice, rice vinegar, and cornstarch. Blend until completely smooth. Pour into a saucepan and cook over high heat until sauce thickens. Whisk periodically to ensure the sauce doesn't burn.

In a large, nonstick wok, cook the carrots, onion, and green and red peppers on high heat for 4 to 5 minutes. The onion should not be cooked all the way to translucency, and the peppers should retain some of their crispness. Add to the wok the yams, tofu, and sauce; stir to combine. Serve over cooked rice.

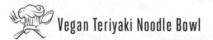 ## Vegan Teriyaki Noodle Bowl

Recipe from Joel Kahn, MD, author of The Plant-Based Solution

Soba is the Japanese name for buckwheat. It usually refers to thin noodles made from buckwheat flour (my preference) or a combination of buckwheat and wheat flours, but it can refer to any thin noodle. They contrast to thick wheat noodles, called *udon*.

Makes 4 servings

Teriyaki Sauce
3 tablespoons rice vinegar
3 tablespoons low-sodium tamari
1 tablespoon low-sodium vegetable broth/stock or water
1 tablespoon natural cane sugar
2 large cloves garlic, grated
1½ teaspoons minced fresh ginger
½ teaspoon red pepper flakes (use less for less heat)
Freshly ground pepper to taste
1 teaspoon potato starch or cornstarch

Noodle Bowl
½ package (4 ounces) soba noodles
2 tablespoons low-sodium vegetable broth/stock or water
3½ cups broccoli florets (½ large bunch)
3 stalks celery, chopped (1¼ cups)
1 large red pepper, thinly sliced (1⅓ cups)
2–3 large carrots, peeled and julienned (1½ cups)
¾–1 cup shelled edamame (optional; thaw if frozen)
3–4 chopped green onions (approximately ½ cup) for
    garnish
Sesame seeds for garnish

Prepare the teriyaki sauce: In a medium bowl, whisk together all the sauce ingredients until combined. Set aside.

For the noodle bowl: Bring a medium pot of water to a boil. Add the soba noodles and reduce heat to medium-high. Cook the noodles according to the package directions. Drain and rinse with cold water; set aside.

Preheat an extra-large skillet or wok over medium-high heat. Add the broth and coat the pan. Add the broccoli florets, celery, and red pepper, and sauté for 7 to 10 minutes, until almost tender. Stir frequently, and reduce heat if necessary to keep the broccoli from burning.

Add the carrots and edamame (if using) to the skillet and sauté for another couple of minutes.

Stir the drained noodles into the stir-fry mixture along with all the teriyaki sauce. Cook for a couple of minutes until the sauce thickens slightly and the carrots soften a bit.

Garnish with green onion and sesame seeds, and serve.

Super-Quick Soba and Veggies

Recipe adapted from Healthy Heart, Healthy Planet *by Dr. Cathi Misquitta and Dr. Rajiv Misquitta*

For this simple and satisfying dish, look for a Korean barbecue sauce with no oil. This product is most likely found in an Asian market, and good ones are sweet and peppery.

Makes 4 servings

1 package (8 ounces) soba noodles
6 heads baby bok choy, washed and cut in half lengthwise
1 onion, chopped into 1-inch pieces

8 ounces baby bella (cremini) mushrooms, halved

⅓ cup Korean barbecue sauce

In a large pot, bring water to a rolling boil and cook the soba noodles according to the package directions. Stir frequently to prevent sticking. When done, drain and rinse.

Meanwhile, in a nonstick wok on high heat, quickly stir-fry the bok choy, onions, and mushrooms for 4 to 5 minutes, or until slightly soft. If there is too much fluid released from the vegetables, sop it up with a paper towel (or two). Remove from heat, add the barbecue sauce, and serve over the noodles.

SOUTHWESTERN AND MEXICAN

Tex-Mex Spaghetti Squash with Black Bean Guacamole

Recipe from Joel Kahn, MD, author of The Plant-Based Solution

This delicious dish is high in protein and fiber while being vegan, gluten-free, grain-free, nut-free, refined sugar–free, and soy-free — not to mention very hearty and filling!

Makes 4 servings

Spaghetti Squash
1 medium spaghetti squash
½ cup low-sodium vegetable broth/stock or water
Pinch of chili powder
Pinch of ground cumin
½ teaspoon dried oregano
½ teaspoon salt
½ teaspoon pepper

Black Bean Guacamole
2 avocados, pitted and flesh scooped out
½ cup diced red onion
1 small tomato, seeded and diced
1 can (15 ounces) black beans, drained and rinsed (or about
    1½ cups cooked beans)
¼ cup chopped cilantro leaves
2 tablespoons fresh lime juice, or to taste
Salt
Pepper
Red pepper flakes

Preheat the oven to 375°F and line a large baking sheet with parchment paper. Slice off the stem of the squash and place the squash cut side down on a cutting board. With a chef's knife, carefully slice through the squash lengthwise to create two long halves. Scoop out the seeds and guts with an ice-cream scoop or large spoon. Brush some broth or water onto the squash and sprinkle with pepper. Place the squash halves cut side down on the baking sheet and roast for 30 to 50 minutes, depending on how large the squash is. When the squash is tender and you can easily scrape the strands with a fork, it's ready. Be sure not to cook it for too long, or it will turn mushy.

While the squash is roasting, prepare the black bean guacamole. In a large bowl, mash the avocado flesh. Fold in the onion, tomato, black beans, and cilantro. Season to taste with lime juice, salt, pepper, and red pepper flakes.

Remove the squash from the oven, flip it over, and scrape the flesh with a fork in long motions down the length of the squash. Do this until you've scraped all the strands off the skin. Stir in the chili powder, cumin, oregano, salt, and pepper. Top the squash with the guacamole and serve warm.

Bean and Wild Rice Burgers with Mashed Sweet Potatoes and Spinach

Recipe from Healthy Heart, Healthy Planet *by Dr. Cathi Misquitta and Dr. Rajiv Misquitta*

This dish is filling enough that you won't miss the bun. If you really want to pick up the burger and bite into it, sandwich it between two crisp, fresh romaine leaves.

Makes 6 to 8 servings

Bean and Wild Rice Burgers

2 cups cooked wild black rice

2 cans (30 ounces) black beans, drained

2 tablespoons no-salt seasoning (such as Mrs. Dash)

1 tablespoon garlic powder

½ teaspoon salt

1 onion, finely diced

Mashed Sweet Potatoes and Spinach

Salt (optional)

1½ pounds sweet potatoes, scrubbed and diced

1 bunch spinach, washed thoroughly and chopped

½ cup almond milk, unsweetened

¼ cup nutritional yeast

Preheat the oven to 350°F. To prepare the burgers, in a food processor with an S-blade, combine the rice, beans, no-salt seasoning, garlic powder, and salt and mix for 1 to 2 minutes. The mixture should retain some texture from the rice and beans but be sticky enough to form into patties. Remove from the food processor and place the mixture in a large bowl. Fold in the diced onion. Line a baking sheet with parchment paper. Form 6 to 8 patties roughly ½ inch thick. Bake for 25 minutes.

Meanwhile, boil water in a large stockpot, adding salt if desired. Add the sweet potatoes and boil for 15 to 20 minutes or until the potatoes fall off a fork when pierced. Before draining, add the spinach and allow it to wilt. This should only take a minute. Drain everything in a colander and transfer to a large bowl or the empty stockpot. Mash the potatoes and spinach, adding the almond milk, nutritional yeast, and any extra salt to taste. Serve immediately, alongside the burgers.

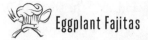 **Eggplant Fajitas**

Recipe adapted from Healthy Heart, Healthy Planet *by Dr. Cathi Misquitta and Dr. Rajiv Misquitta*

When purchasing tortillas for this recipe, be sure to watch the ingredient list. Many tortilla brands contain oil, shortening, or lard (though fat is more commonly included in flour tortillas than corn tortillas). This recipe goes well with a chipotle salsa, but if that is too hot for your palate, feel free to use the salsa of your choice. Many substitutions can be made in this recipe. Instead of gypsy peppers, shimeji mushrooms, and beet greens, you could easily use bell peppers, button mushrooms, and any dark-green leafy vegetable, such as kale, mustard greens, or chard.

Makes 4 servings

1 bunch beet greens
1 large onion, sliced
4 gypsy peppers, seeded and sliced
1 medium globe eggplant, cut into ½-inch cubes
1 ½ cups shimeji mushrooms
¼ cup lime juice
½ teaspoon cumin
½ teaspoon coriander
¼ teaspoon red pepper flakes
½ teaspoon salt
½ bunch cilantro leaves, chopped
Corn tortillas
1 can (15 ounces) black beans or nonfat refried beans
Chipotle or other salsa

Remove the stems from the beet greens and chop the stems into small pieces. Coarsely chop the beet greens. In a large non-stick skillet, cook the onion, peppers, eggplant, beet stems, and mushrooms over medium heat. As the vegetables begin to soften and caramelize, add the lime juice to lift the browning bits and steam the vegetables. Stir in the cumin, coriander, red pepper flakes, salt, and cilantro and cook for 1 minute. Stir in the beet greens until wilted. Remove from heat.

Wrap the tortillas in foil and warm them in the oven, and heat the beans on the stove. Spoon the vegetables into the tortillas, and top with salsa. Serve with the black beans on the side.

Eggplant Mole with Quinoa

Recipe adapted from Healthy Heart, Healthy Planet *by Dr. Cathi Misquitta and Dr. Rajiv Misquitta*

Here's another recipe that showcases fiber-rich, heart-healthy eggplant, this time in a healthy twist on mole, the beloved traditional Mexican sauce.

Makes 4 servings

Vegetables and Quinoa
1 globe eggplant, halved lengthwise and sliced into
    ½-inch pieces
Salt
2 cups low-sodium vegetable broth/stock or water
1 cup quinoa
1 small mild to medium chili pepper (such as serrano), diced

1 onion, diced

1 bunch spinach, washed thoroughly and chopped

2 ears corn, kernels removed, or 1 cup frozen or drained
    canned corn

Corn tortillas

1 can (15 ounces) nonfat refried black beans

Mole

½ onion, finely diced

1 small mild to medium chili pepper (such as serrano),
    finely diced

½ apple, finely diced

2 cloves garlic, finely diced

3 tablespoons lemon juice

6 ounces tomato paste

¼ cup fresh cilantro, chopped

1 tablespoon cocoa powder

1½ teaspoons cumin

½ teaspoon salt

1½ cups unsweetened almond milk

Preheat the oven to 400°F. Line a baking sheet with parchment paper. Place the eggplant slices on the parchment paper, sprinkle with a little salt, and bake for 25 minutes. Set aside.

Meanwhile, in a large pot, bring the vegetable stock to a boil, then add the quinoa, pepper, and onion and reduce heat to medium-low. Cover and simmer for 15 minutes. Fold in the spinach and corn kernels. Cover and simmer until all the stock is absorbed by the quinoa.

Wrap the tortillas in foil and warm them in the oven, and heat the beans, either on the stove or in the microwave.

While the quinoa is cooking, make the mole. In a large dry saucepan, cook the onion, pepper, apple, and garlic, stirring, until they begin to caramelize. Reduce the heat and add the lemon juice, tomato paste, cilantro, cocoa, cumin, and salt. Once these are combined, add the almond milk and whisk until it is fully incorporated.

To serve, place one tortilla on each plate. In thirds on each tortilla, add the eggplant, quinoa, and beans. Spoon a generous quantity of mole on the eggplant and drizzle on the quinoa and beans.

PASTA

Vegan Oil-Free Pasta and Veggies

Recipe from Joel Kahn, MD, author of The Plant-Based Solution

For this basic but tasty dish, instead of whole-wheat pasta, you can use brown-rice pasta, which is very healthy! Any kind of tomatoes or olives will work.

Makes 4 servings

1 small head broccoli, cut into 10 florets
1 carrot, thinly sliced
½ pound whole-wheat pasta
5 tomatoes, chopped or pureed
Spices to taste (such as Italian seasoning mix, fresh-cut
     parsley, and/or coriander)
Pepper to taste
7 olives, pitted and chopped
Fresh spinach
5–6 small mushrooms, or 2–3 large ones, sliced

Put a pot of water on the stove and bring to a boil.

While the water is heating, heat a thick-bottomed pan for 30 seconds on high, and then add the broccoli and carrots. Turn the heat to medium-low and toss the vegetables in the pan for 2 minutes. Stir continuously to make sure they don't burn.

Once the water is boiling, add the pasta, and cook until al dente according to the package directions.

Add the tomatoes, spices, and pepper to the broccoli and carrots, and cook on low for 5 minutes, stirring continuously. Finally, add the olives, as many spinach leaves as you like, and the mushrooms, and cook on medium for 3 to 5 more minutes, stirring continuously. Taste the vegetable mixture and adjust the seasonings as necessary. When the pasta is ready, drain it. Add the pasta to the vegetables and mix well. Serve immediately.

Quick-and-Easy Creamy Tomato Mushroom Pasta

Recipe from Joel Kahn, MD, author of The Plant-Based Solution

Nutritional yeast is a flavorful vegan cheese alternative that provides a creamy consistency while adding its unique savory flavor to this yummy pasta dish. Whole-wheat and brown-rice pastas both work well here.

Makes 4 servings

1 small sweet onion, diced
3 cloves garlic, minced
1 teaspoon low-sodium vegetable broth/stock or water
½ pound whole-grain pasta
8 ounces mushrooms, sliced (about 2–3 cups)
1 can (15 ounces) diced tomatoes
¾ cup chopped fresh basil leaves
¼–⅓ cup nutritional yeast
1½ tablespoons tomato paste
1 teaspoon dried oregano

¼ teaspoon dried thyme
¼ teaspoon red pepper flakes (optional)
Salt

Put a pot of water on the stove and bring to a boil.

While the water is heating, heat a large skillet or wok over medium heat. Sauté the onion and garlic in the broth or water for about 5 minutes, or until translucent.

Once the water is boiling, add the pasta, and cook until al dente according to the package directions.

Stir the sliced mushrooms and your desired amount of diced tomatoes into the onions and garlic, and cook for another 8 to 10 minutes over medium-high heat, until some of the tomato water cooks off.

Stir in the basil, nutritional yeast (use more or less as you desire), tomato paste, oregano, thyme, and red pepper flakes, if using. Add salt to taste. Simmer for another 5 minutes or so and add more seasonings as desired.

Drain the pasta and put it back into the pot. Stir the sauce into the pasta, reheat if needed, and serve immediately.

Pasta and Greens with Smoky Butternut Squash Sauce

Recipe from Joel Kahn, MD, author of The Plant-Based Solution

Thanks to the cashews and nutritional yeast, you won't miss cheese in this pasta at all! If you have any leftover cooked veggies in the fridge, they can find a home here.

Makes 4 servings

¼ cup raw cashews

1 (3½–4-pound) butternut squash, peeled, seeded, and diced
　　(or two 1-pound packages chopped squash)

¾ cup water

2 cloves garlic

2 tablespoons nutritional yeast (optional)

1 tablespoon fresh lemon juice

½ teaspoon onion powder

½ teaspoon smoked paprika

¼ teaspoon chili powder

Hot sauce

½ pound whole-grain mini-shell or macaroni pasta

Broccoli, kale, or other vegetables (optional)

Put the cashews in a small bowl and cover with water. Soak overnight or for at least 3 hours, until soft and plump. Drain and rinse before use.

Preheat the oven to 425°F and line a baking sheet with parchment paper. Spread out the chopped squash on the sheet. Roast for 30 to 40 minutes, flipping once halfway through baking, until the squash is fork-tender. Let cool for at least 5 minutes.

In a high-speed blender, combine the soaked and drained cashews, water, garlic, nutritional yeast (if using), lemon juice, onion powder, paprika, chili powder, and 2 cups of cooked squash. Blend on high until smooth. Add the hot sauce to taste and blend again.

Cook the pasta until al dente according to the package directions. If using broccoli, kale, or other vegetables, cook them while the pasta is cooking, either steaming or sautéing for 5 to 10 minutes over medium heat. Or use leftover cooked veggies.

When the pasta is cooked and drained, return it to the pot. Pour on the sauce and stir to combine. Stir in the cooked vegetables, if using. If needed, reheat over medium heat, and serve immediately.

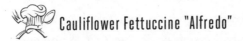

Cauliflower Fettuccine "Alfredo"

Recipe from Joel Kahn, MD, author of The Plant-Based Solution

This take on a traditional favorite incorporates cauliflower to pack in the phytochemicals. You can also add cooked peas, sautéed spinach, roasted broccoli, or any other favorite vegetables. These work very nicely to turbocharge the nutritional benefits!

Makes 4 servings

1 medium head cauliflower, cut into 4 heaping cups of florets
1 tablespoon low-sodium vegetable broth/stock or water
1 tablespoon minced garlic
½ cup unsweetened and unflavored almond milk (or nondairy milk of choice)
¼ cup nutritional yeast
1 tablespoon fresh lemon juice
½ teaspoon onion powder
¼–½ teaspoon garlic powder
¼–½ teaspoon pepper, and to taste
½ pound whole-grain fettuccine
Peas, spinach, or broccoli (optional)
Pepper
Minced fresh parsley for garnish

In a large pot, cover the cauliflower florets with water. Bring to a low boil. Once boiling, cook for another 3 to 7 minutes until fork-tender. Drain.

Meanwhile, in a skillet, combine the broth and garlic and sauté over low heat for 4 to 5 minutes, until the garlic is softened and fragrant but not browned.

In a high-speed blender, combine the cooked cauliflower, sautéed garlic, milk, nutritional yeast, lemon juice, onion powder, garlic powder, and pepper. Blend until a super-smooth sauce forms. To make sure it's really smooth, don't be afraid to let the blender run for a minute or so. Set the sauce aside.

Bring a large pot of water to a boil. Cook the pasta according to the package instructions. While the pasta is cooking, cook the peas, sauté the spinach, or roast the broccoli. Drain the pasta and return it to the pot.

Add the cauliflower sauce and stir to combine. If using peas, spinach, or broccoli, add those to the pot. Warm over low-medium heat if necessary. Season with pepper, garnish with parsley, and serve.

Roasted Romanesco Cauliflower and Asparagus Pasta

Recipe adapted from Healthy Heart, Healthy Planet *by Dr. Cathi Misquitta and Dr. Rajiv Misquitta*

Romanesco cauliflower (also known as Romanesco broccoli or just Romanesco) is a cruciferous vegetable native to Italy that has a crunchier texture and milder flavor than cauliflower. Its appearance is fascinating because it's a natural manifestation of a fractal, an infinitely repeating mathematical shape. Bragg's

Liquid Aminos, a beloved healthy alternative to soy sauce, can be found at natural-food stores.

Makes 4 servings

1 head Romanesco cauliflower, florets separated and cut in half
1 package (16 ounces) organic silken tofu
½ cup lemon juice
1 tablespoon Bragg's Liquid Aminos
⅓ cup nutritional yeast
½ cup unsweetened almond milk
1 teaspoon minced fresh rosemary
½ pound whole-wheat rotini
1 onion, diced
2 cloves garlic, diced
8 ounces baby bella (cremini) mushrooms, sliced
¼ cup dry white wine (such as chardonnay)
1 bunch asparagus, cut diagonally into ½-inch-thick pieces

Preheat the oven to 350°F. Place the cauliflower florets flat side down on a nonstick baking sheet and bake for 30 minutes.

While the cauliflower is roasting, in a blender, combine the tofu, lemon juice, Bragg's Liquid Aminos, nutritional yeast, almond milk, and rosemary, and blend until smooth.

Bring a pot of water to a boil, and cook the pasta according to the package directions.

Meanwhile, in a large dry nonstick skillet sauté the onion, garlic, and mushrooms over medium heat until caramelized, about 10 minutes, then stir in the white wine. Cook for another minute or 2, until the wine evaporates.

Add the tofu mixture to the mushrooms and onions and simmer for another 5 minutes.

In a separate shallow skillet, boil the asparagus for 3 to 5 minutes, until al dente. A fork inserted should lightly cling to the asparagus, and the asparagus should fall off easily with a small shake; be careful not to overcook it.

To assemble, place pasta in each bowl, cover with the sauce, and then top with the asparagus and cauliflower.

VEGGIE SIDES

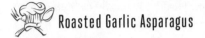 **Roasted Garlic Asparagus**

Recipe adapted from Healthy Heart, Healthy Planet *by Dr. Cathi Misquitta and Dr. Rajiv Misquitta*

Asparagus is high in dietary fiber to help you feel full, plus folate and other vitamins and minerals. It's a spring vegetable with a short in-season window — get it locally while you can!

Makes 6 servings

½ cup extra-virgin olive oil
8 cloves fresh garlic, minced
1 teaspoon onion powder
2 tablespoons fresh finely chopped parsley
2 pounds thin asparagus, ends trimmed
Coarse sea salt
Freshly ground pepper

Preheat the oven to 400°F. Line a large rimmed baking sheet with parchment paper. Set aside.

In a small saucepan, heat the oil, garlic, onion powder, and parsley on medium-low heat. Cook for 3 minutes, until the garlic mixture is fragrant but not browned.

Spread the asparagus in a single layer on the prepared pan. Lightly sprinkle with the salt and pepper. Drizzle on the garlic-oil mixture.

Roast for 8 to 10 minutes, until the asparagus are bright green; do not overcook. Transfer to a platter and serve hot.

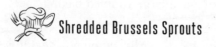

Roasted Broccoli with Garlic

Recipe adapted from Healthy Heart, Healthy Planet *by Dr. Cathi Misquitta and Dr. Rajiv Misquitta*

Broccoli just might be the king of all superfoods.

Makes 4 servings

1 bunch broccoli (about 1½ pounds), cut into florets
2 tablespoons extra-virgin olive oil
3 cloves garlic, sliced
Kosher salt
Freshly ground pepper

In a skillet over medium heat, toss the broccoli florets with the olive oil, garlic, salt, and pepper. Spread the florets out in the pan and then roast, without stirring, until the edges are slightly crispy and the stems are crisp-tender, about 7 to 10 minutes. Then, shake to stir the contents of the pan once and leave on medium heat for 5 more minutes. Serve warm.

Shredded Brussels Sprouts

Recipe adapted from Eat to Live Cookbook *by Joel Fuhrman, MD*

Yet another wonderful cruciferous vegetable! In this recipe, prepare the toasted walnuts ahead: In a small skillet over medium heat, cook for 2 to 3 minutes until lightly toasted.

Makes 4 servings

2 tablespoons water, plus more as needed

2 cloves garlic, chopped

¾ pound Brussels sprouts, cut into ⅛-inch ribbons

¼ cup chopped toasted walnuts (see note above)

2 tablespoons raisins or currants

1 tablespoon nutritional yeast

Freshly ground pepper

In a large skillet, heat the water. Add the garlic and sauté for 1 minute. Add the shredded Brussels sprouts and cook for 2 to 3 minutes, until warm and slightly wilted. Add a small amount of additional water if needed to prevent from sticking.

Remove from heat and toss with the walnuts, raisins or currants, and nutritional yeast. Season with pepper.

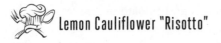 ## Lemon Cauliflower "Risotto"

Recipe adapted from Eat to Live Cookbook *by Joel Fuhrman, MD*

Riced cauliflower is getting increasingly popular because it offers the heartiness of rice or couscous while being a low-calorie superfood. If you need guidance on how to "rice" it, search online for a tutorial or video.

Makes 4 servings

2–3 tablespoons water

½ onion, diced

2 cloves garlic, finely chopped

½ cup low-sodium or no-salt-added vegetable broth

6 cups very finely chopped (riced) cauliflower florets
Juice and zest of ½ organic lemon
1 cup sliced roasted red bell peppers
1 tablespoon nutritional yeast
2 cups finely sliced spinach
4 tablespoons raw almond butter
2 tablespoons sliced chives, divided
2 tablespoons chopped raw almonds

In a large pot or sauté pan, heat 2 to 3 tablespoons of water. Add the onion and garlic, and sauté, stirring often, until tender, about 4 minutes.

Add the vegetable broth and cauliflower, and sauté for 3 minutes. Add the lemon juice and zest, roasted red peppers, nutritional yeast, spinach, almond butter, and 1 tablespoon of the chives. Cook for 3 more minutes or until the cauliflower is al dente. Sprinkle the almonds and remaining chives over the risotto. Serve immediately.

Conclusion

The question isn't who is going to let me; it's who is going to stop me.

— AYN RAND

Close your eyes for a moment and think of someone you really care about, such as a child, a spouse, a loving parent, or even a pet. Think of a beautiful experience — an image, a place, a piece of soothing music — or a situation where you truly improved someone's life. How does that feel? Are you experiencing a visceral, gratifying physical response? Even though you are not having that experience right now, just the thought of it evokes a pleasurable response. This feeling of love and beauty, and feeling connected to a life of purpose and meaning, has helped people survive the most harrowing of circumstances.

Ask Yourself Why

When I see new patients, I often ask them why they came to see me. The usual initial response is something along the lines of "because I want to lose weight" or "to improve my health."

However, I keep asking the question, and the third or fourth time, people get more specific: They want to move more freely without feeling winded, or they want to travel to another part of the world or to be alive for an important family event, such as a grandchild's wedding. Eventually, often after five repetitions, patients answer the question why with their deepest reasons for seeking a change — to become a significant factor in someone's life; to love and be loved; to enjoy the beautiful experiences of life; to grow, learn, and contribute; to leave behind a meaningful legacy.

Of the thousands of books you could have picked up, you chose this one, and there is a very good reason you are still reading. You are on Earth for a very specific purpose, and your job is to find it. In the words of Pablo Picasso, "The meaning of life is to find your gift. The purpose of life is to give it away."

Losing weight and achieving good health are, like wealth, merely a means to an end. The end is what is revealed upon asking the question why until you discover your deepest reasons. This almost always relates to loving and being loved, to doing things that matter, and to living a life that makes a positive difference.

You have embarked on a project of grand scale, a journey to take back control of your destiny in the universe, to change the trajectory of the rest of your life. This takes a courageous commitment to your deeply held convictions. It takes choosing to live with integrity and vision so that your thoughts, speech, and actions are in complete alignment.

You will have successes that will serve as landmarks. These successes, as small as they may seem at the time, call for celebration. You will also slip up from time to time. Backslides are an inevitable part of the process and should not be met with surprise or be the cause of prolonged remorse. Having a supportive social network, a cheerleading team of friends who can help you without judgment, can help you stay accountable and on track. Much like navigating a huge ship, you will need to make adjustments to your course when needed. The most important requirement is an unfaltering commitment to your end goals and the deep-rooted reasons why you started on this journey in the first place, whatever those are.

Already within you reside all the tools you need to achieve your goals, your mission, and your purpose in life. You might need to upgrade your "software" if your current system runs on limiting beliefs and negative thoughts, attitudes, and emotions. This will need to be replaced with confidence and belief in yourself and in your body's own unlimited capacity to heal and flourish.

So, once again, explore your unique reason for embarking on this journey. Ask yourself why five times, or as many times as you need to discover your deepest reasons. Then, if you haven't already, fill out appendix 2, "Ten Reasons Why I Want to Achieve Turbo Metabolism." Once you are very clear about why you need to change, you can initiate massive action. As long as you never lose sight of why you started the journey to Turbo Metabolism, you will have plenty of reasons to celebrate all the successes along the way. Always keep in mind: You can fulfill your deepest primal needs and your wildest dreams.

You may need to rewrite the story you have been telling yourself about your predestined fate into a story where you have the power to harness nature's power of healing, health, and vitality. Success comes when you combine this with the hard work and discipline of habit change: Automation of the environment leads to liberation, so that you can spend your

time and energy on the things that really matter. The rest is
minor details.

By following the principles and instructions outlined in this
book, you can create a new environment where the right choice
becomes the easy choice 100 percent of the time. You can reset
your world so that your choices will help you fulfill your personal goals and meet your deepest needs in the short time you
have on this planet.

Ask yourself: *Why am I here? What is it that I really want
to do in my life? How am I going to get from where I am to where
I want to be?*

Then, take the first step. Remember, progress — not perfection — is the goal. As you see your results, both positive and
negative, you will grow. As you grow, you will feel rewarded.
Results lead to growth, and growth provides rewards.

I wish you the best of luck on your journey. May you add
many years to your life and much life to your years.

Putting It All Together

By now, you should have a basic understanding of how various
lifestyle factors can contribute significantly to chronic metabolic diseases, including obesity, diabetes, heart attacks, strokes,
and cancer. These negative factors include poor diet and nutrition; sleep deprivation; lack of exercise; lack of emotional resilience, which manifests as out-of-control stress; missing social
support; and prolonged exposure to environmental toxins, both
physical and psychological.

You might have realized that a lot of our problems are from
pretending to have forgotten what we knew to be true a long
time ago: It is good to eat mostly vegetables, to be and play
outside with friends in the sun, to match our body and sleep

rhythms with the sun's cycle, and to not fret about things that are beyond our control.

You understand that making critical changes to these life-style factors can prevent or reverse disease. Hopefully, you are now motivated enough to implement your own program of changes in consultation with your physician, starting with small changes, while setting up the environment to help you succeed.

The evidence is solid and incontrovertible. Metabolic diseases, prediabetes, diabetes, and even coronary artery disease (associated with being overweight or obese) are absolutely preventable and reversible. They should no longer be thought of as chronic, progressive, and debilitating conditions. They are not your destiny.

Many modern lifestyle factors cause insulin resistance, but overeating is the worst. It's so easy to succumb to a diet of processed poisons masquerading as food and loaded with refined carbs such as sugar and corn syrup, beer and wine, and fast food loaded with unhealthy trans and saturated animal fats. There is no fiber in most processed foods, and there is a serious lack of micronutrients. We are bombarded with environmental toxins that are poisoning our mitochondria and dumb ideas that are poisoning our minds. On top of that, we are increasingly sedentary, overstressed, lonely, and sleep deprived.

When we begin to understand the root causes of these imbalances, we can eliminate them. It should be clear that it is as important to eliminate the things that make us weak and sick as it is to add in the things that can help heal and make us stronger. As our understanding of the science shifts, the paradigm shifts.

Fear of sickness and death can be an initial trigger, but sustained change means emotional buy-in to a positive outcome and massive action. This means setting up your immediate environment for success, including the physical (your kitchen, refrigerator, snack drawer); the social (gaining the support of people close to you); and the psychological (your commitment to positive choices and positive thinking). Creating an environment where healthy choices come naturally is critical. It definitely takes work, such as planning to navigate around parties, special occasions, and restaurant menus. But the rewards are well worth the effort.

Thousands of people before you have regained their well-being, strength, and vitality. And so can you. When you learn from credible sources, and then *own* the knowledge and set up your physical, social, and psychological environments for success, you can move from reluctant action (or compliance) to a lifelong commitment. As a bonus, you'll look and feel much better, too!

Fun, freedom, and joy — autonomy, mastery, and purpose — are the real motivators for change, and I sincerely hope you feel that your life is noticeably more enjoyable as you make better dietary and lifestyle choices. I hope you can approach life with energy, enthusiasm, gusto, and passion, so that when you are invited to the next adventure you say, "Yes, bring it on!" instead of, "No, thanks, I don't think I can do that."

Positive reinforcement from feeling better also leads to permanent change as it becomes more and more self-motivating. Ultimately, self-motivation is even more powerful than the compliments you receive from others when your clothes fit so much better. Slipups are inevitable; just jump back on the plan as soon as possible. Remember, the motto is "progress, not perfection."

There are no black-and-white rules about choices; it's all

about understanding the wisdom of the body, paying attention to the signals that you receive from your body and mind, and making the best choices every day. It's about doing those things that make you stronger, about feeding the "superhero" within, and dodging the things that make you weak, tired, sick, and fat. This journey requires mindful attention. Focus on putting forward your best self every moment of every day so that you can overcome the fear, inhibitions, and obstacles that are in the way of the fulfillment of your mission, the achievement of the purpose of your existence.

Whenever a "trash food" presents itself, just consider: Which do you prefer, the toxic substances that feed disease and that stress you out or the nourishing, enriching, healing ones that improve your life?

The real point isn't longevity. What do you gain adding years to your life if those years are spent drooling in a rocking chair? The point is adding life to your years. It's about enjoying yourself for as long as you can. How much life would you like in your remaining years? Do you want to fulfill your vision, your life's mission and purpose, your wildest dreams? You have the power to decide.

The choice is yours.

TURBO METABOLISM RULES TO LIVE BY

- Find your reasons why.
- Food is medicine: Follow a low-glycemic, nutrient-dense, plant-rich diet.
- Increase insulin sensitivity to get your insulin levels down: This translates to less hunger and more fat burn.
- Eliminate toxins.

- Hydrate.
- Sleep is the force multiplier.
- Move naturally and activate large muscles.
- Build emotional resilience, so you bounce back quickly from setbacks.
- Harness the power of habits, so good choices are automatic.
- Set up the environment for success.
- Invest in social connections and relationships.
- Believe in yourself: Know that you can do it.

Dr. Vij's Ten Commandments for Optimal Wellness

1. Thou shalt stop eating flour and sugar products, especially high-fructose corn syrup.
2. Thou shalt not consume liquid calories, like those in soft drinks, juice drinks, and mixed drinks; drink water instead.
3. Thou shalt stop eating all processed junk and packaged foods.
4. Thou shalt avoid unhealthy fats, such as trans and hydrogenated fats.
5. Thou shalt eat plenty of fiber (at least fifty grams a day).
6. Thou shalt eat balanced meals — healthy proteins (tofu, peas, seaweed, nuts, seeds, beans, and occasionally small wild fish, organic chicken, and organic eggs), healthy carbohydrates (vegetables, fruit, beans, and whole grains), and healthy fats (nuts and seeds, avocados, olive oil, and fish oil) — which slows the rate of sugar uptake from the gut.
7. Thou shalt eat lots of vegetables and more modest amounts of fruit, but avoid especially sugary fruit (bananas, pineapples, kiwi, oranges).
8. Thou shalt get an "oil change" — eat more omega-3 oils to fix cell membranes so that they can more readily receive messages from insulin.
9. Thou shalt move your body through regular exercise, so that your cells work better, respond to insulin better, and burn sugar faster.
10. Thou shalt relax! Stress reduction and restful sleep greatly improve blood-sugar control.

APPENDIX TWO

Ten Reasons Why I Want to Achieve Turbo Metabolism

On a sheet of paper or in a journal, write down ten personal goals and desires for improving your health and reaching Turbo Metabolism. Take your time and give the reasons some thought before writing. These ten reasons should be specific, rather than general, and reflect your genuine, unique motivations, not what you think would please others. Dig deep to express what really motivates you: loving others and being loved; beautiful experiences; opportunities for learning, growth, and contribution, and so on.

Once you're done, you will use this list as your "personal motivator." Each day, several times a day, take a few moments to thoughtfully read through this list. This is called mental programming. Share your ten reasons with friends and even your doctor, who might retain it in your medical file. Make a copy and carry it with you at all times. You could take a photograph with your phone or transfer your list onto a three-by-five card, whichever is more convenient.

Make a promise to yourself now: "I will read the entire list whenever I am confronted with a difficult food situation." Reading the list will reinforce your personal commitment to take control of your health and self-esteem.

Three-Level Exercise Program

If you're ready for a more robust exercise program than the basic, four-month program I offer in chapter 6, try this. This program has three levels, and each level should be followed for at least one month. How fast you proceed is up to you — take longer with each level if you wish. The program is designed to build gradually over time, so that your workouts steadily increase in frequency, intensity, and time (or FIT). Here I provide more specific guidance for how to structure your workout and what to do, but as mentioned before, tailor these suggestions to fit your needs and preferences. Listen to your body, consult your doctor, and adjust as necessary to avoid exhaustion and injury.

Many of these exercises specify using hand weights. Most gyms have these, or you can buy them. If you don't have hand weights, modify the exercises as you wish to work the same muscle groups. In addition, if you are unfamiliar with any of the exercises, search the exercise names online or ask a trainer. Again, when unsure, substitute an exercise that is familiar for you.

Exercise Logs

Each month, keep track of which days you exercise and for how long, using an exercise log. I also suggest weighing yourself at the beginning and end of each month, as well as measuring your percentage of body fat at the beginning and end of each month. Inexpensive body-fat calipers are easy to find and to use. Try to steadily improve the frequency, intensity, and time of your workouts, which you can track with your log.

Below, I've included an example of a simple log; you can also search online for "exercise log" if you'd like to download a printable version, or use your favorite app.

Sample Exercise Log

Month: _____

Starting weight: _____   Ending weight: _____

Starting percentage body fat: _____

Ending percentage body fat: _____

Date	Type of exercise/ activity	Effort (high, moderate, or light)	Total minutes	How I felt

Exercise Level I

Before every workout, always take five minutes to warm up and stretch. Make sure to rest for a minute or two in between each set of repetitions. Finally, hydrate well, before, during, and after.

Level I frequency: Exercise three days per week. If you exercise only two days one week, then exercise four days the next week.

Level I duration: Exercise a minimum of twenty minutes each time, progressing to thirty minutes by the end of four weeks.

Level I warm-up: Five minutes of jumping jacks.

Level I exercises: Follow the sequence below. If using hand weights, always start with the lightest weights and increase the weight only when the weight you're using becomes easy. If you finish this sequence in less than fifteen minutes, begin again, and do as much of another repetition of the sequence as you have time for.

Target	Number of repetitions	Weight
Squats	10	5–10 pounds
Triceps curls	10	2–5 pounds
Arm raises (lateral and front)	10	5–10 pounds
Biceps curls	10	5–10 pounds
Crunches	10	None
Wall presses	10	None

Exercise Level II

Before every workout, always take five minutes to warm up and stretch. Make sure to rest for a minute or two in between each set of repetitions. Finally, hydrate well, before, during, and after.

Level II frequency: Exercise four days per week. If you exercise only three days one week, then exercise five days the next week.

Level II duration: Exercise a minimum of thirty minutes each time, progressing to forty minutes by the end of four weeks.

Level II warm-up: Five minutes of jumping jacks.

Level II exercises: Follow the sequence below. If using hand weights, always start with the lightest weights and increase the weight only when the weight you're using becomes easy. If you finish this sequence in less than twenty-five minutes, begin again, and do as much of another repetition of the sequence as you have time for.

Target	Number of repetitions	Weight
Squats	10–15	5–12 pounds
Triceps curls	10–15	5–8 pounds
Arm raises (lateral and front)	10–15	5–12 pounds
Biceps curls	10–15	5–12 pounds
Romanian dead lift	10–15	5–12 pounds

Exercise Level III

Before every workout, always take five minutes to warm up and stretch. Make sure to rest for a minute or two in between each set of repetitions. Finally, hydrate well, before, during, and after.

Level III frequency: Exercise five days per week. If you exercise only four days one week, then exercise six days the next week.

Level III duration: Exercise a minimum of forty minutes each time, progressing to sixty minutes by the end of four weeks.

Level III warm-up: Five minutes of burpees and/or jumping jacks.

Level III exercises: Follow the sequence below. Do three sets of repetitions of each exercise, and after each of these sets, do jumping jacks for thirty seconds. Rest for two to three minutes after completing each type of exercise. If using hand weights, always start with the lightest weights and increase the weight only when the weight you're using becomes easy. If you finish this sequence in less than thirty-five minutes, begin again, and do as much of another repetition of the sequence as you have time for.

Target	Number of repetitions (in three sets)	Weight
Squats	10 / 10 / 8	10–12 pounds
Triceps curls	10 / 10 / 8	8–10 pounds
Arm raises (lateral and front)	10 / 10 / 8	8–10 pounds
Biceps curls	10 / 10 / 8	10–12 pounds
Romanian dead lift	10 / 10 / 8	10–12 pounds

Glycemic Index of Foods

The glycemic index (GI) is the value assigned to foods based on how quickly those foods cause increases in blood sugar. Thus the GI of pure glucose would be 100.

Food Group	Very Low GI (<20)
Vegetables	Most nonstarchy vegetables, including: asparagus, avocados, beet greens, bell peppers, bok choy, broccoli, Brussels sprouts, cabbage, cauliflower, celery, collard greens, cucumbers, fennel (bulb), green beans, kale, mushrooms (cremini), mustard greens, olives, olive oil, romaine and other lettuce, spinach, summer squash, Swiss chard, tomatoes, turnip greens
Fruits	
Nuts and seeds	Flaxseeds, sesame seeds

	Low GI (21–55)	Medium GI (56–69)	High GI (>70)
	Carrots, eggplant, garlic, green peas, onions, sea vegetables (dulse, kombu, nori), winter squash	Beets, corn, leeks, sweet potatoes	Potatoes
	Apples, bananas, blueberries, cranberries, grapefruit, grapes, kiwi, lemons/limes, oranges, pears, plums, prunes, raspberries, strawberries	Apricots, cantaloupe, figs, papaya, pineapple, raisins, watermelon	
	Almonds, cashews, peanuts, pumpkin seeds, sunflower seeds, walnuts		

Food Group	Very Low GI (<20)
Beans and other legumes	Soybeans, tempeh, tofu
Seafood	Cod, salmon, sardines, shrimp, tuna
Meats*	Beef, grass-fed; chicken, pasture-raised; lamb, grass-fed; turkey, pasture-raised
Dairy products and eggs*	
Grains	
World's healthiest spices and herbs	Black pepper, chili pepper, cilantro, cinnamon, cloves, coriander seeds, cumin seeds, dill, ginger, mustard seeds, oregano, parsley, peppermint, rosemary, sage, thyme, turmeric

* I recommend avoiding animal protein as much as possible, for all the reasons discussed earlier.

	Low GI (21–55)	Medium GI (56–69)	High GI (>70)
	Black beans, chickpeas (garbanzo beans), dried peas, kidney beans, lentils, lima beans, navy beans, pinto beans		
	Scallops		
	Cheese, grass-fed; cow's milk, grass-fed; eggs, pasture-raised; yogurt, grass-fed		
	Barley, brown rice, buckwheat, bulgur, oats, quinoa, rye, whole wheat, wild rice	Millet	White rice

Acknowledgments

I am immensely thankful to my wife, Minnie, for allowing me time and space and tolerating all my obsessions; our parents — Inder and Sneh, and Jaswant and Kartar; my boys, Arjun and Abhay; and my brother, Dr. Neeraj Vij. I am grateful for Sushil, Jennifer, Kevin, Priyanka and Neeraj Jr., Lanee, Danica, little Ollie, and the rest of my cheerleading team.

I am deeply indebted to all my patients and to my colleagues and mentors who have helped shape me into who I am today. I want to first express my gratitude especially to my mentors, Drs. Doug Amis, Neal Barnard, Joel Fuhrman, Mladen Golubic (from the Cleveland Clinic), Joel Kahn, John La Puma, Rajiv Misquitta, Ed Parks, and Sandor Shoichet, who have been a major source of encouragement and positivity.

I am grateful to all my colleagues, especially the following doctors: Devi Banda, Sherilynn Cooke, Jerry Deck, Mark Gullapalli, Lakshmi Mahendran, Muniza Muzaffar, Malalai Nasiri, Deep Patel, Vasantha Ravi Shankar, Ria San Valentin, Rina Shinn, Namrata Sidhu, Dirk Smith, Savitha Sundararaj, Afshan Umair, Surekha Urva, and Jackie Yuen; as well as Dr. Sharon Mowat, Dr. Ken Grullon, and Dr. Mark Hlavac for their support.

I am grateful to my editorial team, including Hal Strauss; my agent, Lisa Hagan; copyeditor Jeff Campbell; proofreader Tanya Fox; and all the great folks at New World Library, especially my editor Georgia Hughes, Kristen Cashman, Kim Corbin, Tona Pearce Myers, and Tracy Cunningham, who helped transform my dream of publishing a book into reality.

Notes

Introduction: Why Turbo Metabolism, and What's in It for Me?

1. "Adult Obesity Facts," Centers for Disease Control and Prevention, last modified August 29, 2017, https://www.cdc.gov/obesity/data/adult.html.
2. Andy Menke et al., "Prevalence of and Trends in Diabetes among Adults in the United States, 1988–2012," *JAMA* 314, no. 10 (2015): 1021, doi:10.1001/jama.2015.10029.
3. Eric Pianin, "US Health Care Costs Surge to 17 Percent of GDP," *Fiscal Times*, December 3, 2015, http://www.thefiscaltimes.com/2015/12/03/Federal-Health-Care-Costs-Surge-17-Percent-GDP.
4. M. K. Hoy, J. D. Goldman, and R. S. Sebastian, "Fruit and Vegetable Intake of US Adults Estimated by Two Methods: What We Eat in America, National Health and Nutrition Examination Survey 2009–2012," *Public Health Nutrition* 19, no. 14 (March 31, 2016): 1–5, https://www.ncbi.nlm.nih.gov/pubmed/27029618.
5. Richard Bach, *Illusions* (New York: Dell Publishing, 1977), 92.

Chapter 1. Metabolic Syndrome: The Root Cause of Chronic Disease

1. A. Onat, "Metabolic Syndrome: Nature, Therapeutic Solutions, and Options," *Expert Opinion on Pharmacotherapy* 12, no. 12 (August 2011): 1887–1900, doi:10.1517/14656566.2011.585462.
2. S. Fröjdö, H. Vidal, and L. Pirola, "Alterations of Insulin Signaling in Type 2 Diabetes: A Review of the Current Evidence from Humans," *Biochimica et Biophysica Acta* 1792, no. 2 (February 2009): 83–92, figure 1, doi:10.1016/j.bbadis.2008.10.019.
3. "Leading Causes of Death," Centers for Disease Control and

Prevention, last modified March 17, 2017, https://www.cdc.gov
/nchs/fastats/leading-causes-of-death.htm.

4. T. Halmos and I. Suba, "Alzheimer's Disease and Diabetes: The
Common Pathogenesis," *Neuropsychopharmacologia Hungarica* 18,
no. 1 (March 2016): 5–19, https://www.ncbi.nlm.nih.gov/pubmed
/27038867.

5. M. Monami et al., "Fasting and Post-prandial Glucose and Diabetic
Complication: A Meta-analysis," *Nutrition, Metabolism, and Cardiovascular Diseases* 23, no. 7 (July 2013): 591–98, doi:10.1016/j.numecd
.2013.03.007.

6. P. G. Cohen, "Aromatase, Adiposity, Aging, and Disease: The
Hypogonadal-Metabolic-Atherogenic-Disease and Aging
Connection," *Medical Hypotheses* 56, no. 6 (June 2001): 702–8,
https://www.ncbi.nlm.nih.gov/pubmed/11399122.

7. Roberta Fontana and Sara Della Torre, "The Deep Correlation between Energy Metabolism and Reproduction: A View on the Effects
of Nutrition for Women Fertility," *Nutrients* 8, no. 2 (February 2016):
87, doi:10.3390/nu8020087.

Chapter 2. A Holistic Approach toward the Treatment and Cure for Diabesity

1. Brian Hodgkinson, *The Essence of Vedanta: The Ancient Wisdom of
Indian Philosophy* (London: Eagle Editions Limited, 2006).

2. B. K. S. Iyengar, *Yoga: The Path to Holistic Health* (New York: DK
Publishing, 2001).

3. David Simon, *The Wisdom of Healing: A Natural Mind Body Program
for Optimal Wellness* (New York: Three Rivers Press, 1997).

Chapter 3. The Nuts and Bolts of Getting Started

1. J. van't Riet et al., "The Importance of Habits in Eating Behaviour:
An Overview and Recommendations for Future Research," *Appetite*
57, no. 3 (December 2011): 585–96, doi:10.1016/j.appet.2011.07.010;
"References to Related Work," BJ Fogg's Behavior Model, http://
www.behaviormodel.org/references.html.

2. S. E. Swithers, A. A. Martin, and T. L. Davidson, "High-Intensity
Sweeteners and Energy Balance," *Physiology & Behavior* 100, no. 1
(April 2010): 55–62, doi:10.1016/j.physbeh.2009.12.021.

3. M. M. Andreatta et al., "Artificial Sweetener Consumption and Urinary Tract Tumors in Cordoba, Argentina," *Preventive Medicine* 47, no. 1 (July 2008): 136–39, doi:10.1016/j.ypmed.2008.03.015.

4. R. Kaaks and A. Lukanova, "Energy Balance and Cancer: The Role of Insulin and Insulin-Like Growth Factor-I," *The Proceedings of the Nutrition Society* 60, no. 1 (February 2001): 91–106, https://www.ncbi.nlm.nih.gov/pubmed/11310428.

5. "Health Concerns about Dairy Products," Physicians Committee for Responsible Medicine, http://www.pcrm.org/health/diets/vegdiets/health-concerns-about-dairy-products.

6. S. Kamiński, A. Cieslińska, and E. Kostyra, "Polymorphism of Bovine Beta-casein and Its Potential Effect on Human Health," *Journal of Applied Genetics* 48, no. 3 (2007): 189–98, doi:10.1007/BF03195213.

7. P. Chatonnet, S. Boutou, and A. Plana, "Contamination of Wines and Spirits by Phthalates: Types of Contaminants Present, Contamination Sources, and Means of Prevention," *Food Additives & Contaminants, Part A, Chemistry, Analysis, Control, Exposure & Risk Assessment* 31, no. 9 (2014): 1605–15, doi:10.1080/19440049.2014.941947.

8. D. W. Lachenmeier et al., "Can Resveratrol in Wine Protect against the Carcinogenicity of Ethanol?: A Probabilistic Dose-Response Assessment," *International Journal of Cancer* 134, no. 1 (January 2014): 144–53, doi:10.1002/ijc.28336.

9. M. Kotepui, "Diet and Risk of Breast Cancer," *Contemporary Oncology* 20, no. 1 (2016): 13–19, doi:10.5114/wo.2014.40560.

10. "Alcohol and Cancer Risk," National Cancer Institute, last modified June 24, 2013, https://www.cancer.gov/about-cancer/causes-prevention/risk/alcohol/alcohol-fact-sheet#q6.

11. M. Stott-Miller, M. L. Neuhouser, and J. L. Stanford, "Consumption of Deep-Fried Foods and Risk of Prostate Cancer," *The Prostate* 73, no. 9 (June 2013): 960–69, doi:10.1002/pros.22643.

12. W. M. Fernando et al., "The Role of Dietary Coconut for the Prevention and Treatment of Alzheimer's Disease: Potential Mechanisms of Action," *British Journal of Nutrition* 114, no. 1 (July 14, 2015): 1–14, doi:10.1017/S0007114515001452.

13. Jim Kwik, "Kwik Brain 001: Learn ANYTHING Faster," Jim Kwik blog, last modified March 30, 2017, http://jimkwik.com/kwik-brain-001.

14. Christine Carter, *The Sweet Spot* (New York: Ballantine Books, 2015).

Chapter 4. Optimal Nutrition for Optimal Health

1. Joel Fuhrman, *Eat to Live* (New York: Little, Brown and Company, 2003).
2. Herbert L. DuPont and James H. Steele, "The Human Health Implication of the Use of Antimicrobial Agents in Animal Feeds," *Veterinary Quarterly* 9, no. 4 (1987): 309–20, doi:10.1080/01652176 .1987.9694119.
3. S. B. Eaton, "The Ancestral Human Diet: What Was It and Should It Be a Paradigm for Contemporary Nutrition?" *Proceedings of the Nutrition Society* 65, no. 1 (February 2006): 1–6, https://www.ncbi .nlm.nih.gov/pubmed/16441938.
4. Andy Menke et al., "Prevalence of and Trends in Diabetes among Adults in the United States, 1988–2012," *JAMA* 314, no. 10 (2015): 1021–29, doi:10.1001/jama.2015.10029.

Chapter 5. Water: The Stuff of Life

1. "Freshwater Crisis," *National Geographic*, http://www.national geographic.com/freshwater/freshwater-crisis.html.
2. Rachel Casiday and Regina Frey, "Nutrients and Solubility," Washington University in St. Louis, last modified January 2001, http://www.chemistry.wustl.edu/~edudev/LabTutorials/Vitamins /vitamins.html.
3. Douglas S. Kalman and Anna Lepeley, "A Review of Hydration," *Strength and Conditioning Journal* 32, no. 2 (April 2010): 56–63, doi:10.1519/SSC.0b013e3181c21172.
4. M. M. Wilson and J. E. Morley, "Impaired Cognitive Function and Mental Performance in Mild Dehydration," *European Journal of Clinical Nutrition* 57, no. 2 (2003): S24–29, doi:10.1038/sj.ejcn.1601898.
5. D. Benton and H. A. Young, "Do Small Differences in Hydration Status Affect Mood and Mental Performance?" *Nutrition Reviews* 73, no. 2 (September 2015): 83–96, doi:10.1093/nutrit/nuv045.
6. S. N. Cheuvront and R. W. Kenefick, "Dehydration: Physiology, Assessment, and Performance Effects," *Comprehensive Physiology* 4, no. 1 (January 2014): 257–85, doi:10.1002/cphy.c130017.

7. R. P. Schwarzenbach et al., "The Challenge of Micropollutants in Aquatic Systems," *Science* 313, no. 5790 (August 25, 2006): 1072–77, doi:10.1126/science.1127291.

8. US Environmental Protection Agency, Safe Drinking Water Hotline, 800-426-4791, https://www.epa.gov/ground-water-and-drinking -water/safe-drinking-water-hotline.

9. "Knowing Where Your Bottled Water Comes From," *Consumer Reports* (July 2012), http://www.consumerreports.org/cro/magazine /2012/07/do-you-know-where-your-bottled-water-comes-from /index.htm.

10. Ibid.

Chapter 6. The Crucial Role of Exercise

1. S. Wang et al., "Curcumin Promotes Browning of White Adipose Tissue in a Norepinephrine-Dependent Way," *Biochemical and Biophysical Research Communications* 466, no. 2 (October 16, 2015): 247–53, doi:10.1016/j.bbrc.2015.09.018.

2. D. T. McMaster et al., "The Development, Retention, and Decay Rates of Strength and Power in Elite Rugby Union, Rugby League, and American Football: A Systematic Review," *Sports Medicine* 43, no. 5 (May 2013): 367–84, doi:10.1007/s40279-013-0031-3.

3. F. J. Penedo and J. R. Dahn, "Exercise and Well-Being: A Review of Mental and Physical Health Benefits Associated with Physical Activity," *Current Opinion in Psychiatry* 18, no. 2 (March 2005): 189–93, https://www.ncbi.nlm.nih.gov/pubmed/16639173.

4. S. Klamroth et al., "Effects of Exercise Therapy on Postural Instability in Parkinson Disease: A Meta-analysis," *Journal of Neurologic Physical Therapy* 40, no. 1 (January 2016): 3–14, doi:10.1097/NPT .0000000000000117.

Chapter 7. Control Stress Before It Controls You

1. T. H. Holmes and R. H. Rahe, "The Social Readjustment Rating Scale," *Journal of Psychosomatic Research* 11, no. 2 (August 1967): 213–18, https://www.ncbi.nlm.nih.gov/pubmed/6059863.

2. Robert Sapolsky, *Why Zebras Don't Get Ulcers* (New York: Henry Holt and Company, 1994).

3. Yang Claire Yang et al., "Social Relationships and Physiological

Determinants of Longevity across the Human Life Span," *Proceedings of the National Academy of Sciences* 113, no. 3, (January 2016): 578–83, doi:10.1073/pnas.1511085112.

4. B. Egolf, J. Lasker, S. Wolf, and L. Potvin, "The Roseto Effect: A 50-Year Comparison of Mortality Rates," *American Journal of Public Health* 82, no. 8 (August 1992): 1089–92.

5. W.-X. Zhou, D. Sornette, R. A. Hill, and R. I. M. Dunbar, "Discrete Hierarchical Organization of Social Group Sizes," *Proceedings of the Royal Society B* 272, no. 1561 (February 22, 2005): 439–44, doi: 10.1098/rspb.2004.2970.

6. R. A. Emmons and M. E. McCullough, "Counting Blessings Versus Burdens: An Experimental Investigation of Gratitude and Subjective Well-Being in Daily Life," *Journal of Personality and Social Psychology* 84, no. 2 (February 2003): 377–89; Sonja Lyubomirsky, *The How of Happiness* (New York: Penguin, 2007), 90–91: "One group of participants was asked to write down five things for which they were thankful...once a week for ten weeks.... Control groups...were asked to think about either five daily hassles or five major events.... Relative to the control groups, those [who expressed gratitude] tended to feel more optimistic and more satisfied with their lives. Even their health received a boost; they reported fewer physical symptoms (such as headache, acne, coughing, or nausea) and more time spent exercising.... These investigations show for the first time that expressions of gratitude are causally linked to the mental and physical health rewards that we have seen."

7. Fred Bryant, "Savoring Beliefs Inventory (SBI): A Scale for Measuring Beliefs about Savoring," *Journal of Mental Health* 12, no. 2 (2003): 175–96.

8. Mika Kivimäki et al., "Work Stress and Risk of Cardiovascular Mortality: Prospective Cohort Study of Industrial Employees," *BMJ* 325, no. 7369 (October 2002): 857, https://www.ncbi.nlm.nih.gov/pubmed/12386034.

9. Thich Nhat Hanh, *Stepping into Freedom: An Introduction to Monastic Training* (Berkeley, CA: Parallax Press, 1997).

10. Martin Luther, *Faith Alone: A Daily Devotional*, ed. James C. Galvin (Grand Rapids, MI: Zondervan, 2005), 67.

11. Jiddu Krishnamurti, *What Are You Doing with Your Life?* (Ojai, CA: Krishnamurti Publications of America, 2001), 20.

12. David Simon, *The Wisdom of Healing: A Natural Mind-Body Program for Optimal Wellness* (New York: Three Rivers Press, 1997), 223.

13. Simon, *Wisdom of Healing*; "Body Intelligence Techniques, BITS," *The Spiritual Journalist*, posted June 17, 2012, http://thespiritual journalist.blogspot.com/2012/06/body-intelligence-techniques -bits.html.

14. B. Wansink, "Environmental Factors that Increase the Food Intake and Consumption Volume of Unknowing Consumers," *Annual Review of Nutrition* 24 (2004): 455–79, doi:10.1146/annurev.nutr .24.012003.132140.

15. Elisha Goldstein, PhD, "The STOP Practice (Stop, Take a Breath, Observe, Proceed)," accessed September 17, 2017, http://elisha goldstein.com/videos/the-stop-practice.

16. Jonathan M. Wong et al., "Hostility, Health Behaviors, and Risk of Recurrent Events in Patients with Stable Coronary Heart Disease: Findings from the Heart and Soul Study," *Journal of the American Heart Association* 2, no. 5 (October 2013): e000052, doi:10.1161 /JAHA.113.000052.

17. Meyer Friedman and Ray H. Rosenman, "Association of Specific Overt Behavior Pattern with Blood and Cardiovascular Findings: Blood Cholesterol Level, Blood Clotting Time, Incidence of Arcus Senilis, and Clinical Coronary Artery Disease," *JAMA* 169, no. 12 (1959): 1286–96, doi:10.1001/jama.1959.03000290012005.

18. J. C. Barefoot, W. G. Dahlstrom, and R. B. Williams Jr., "Hostility, CHD Incidence, and Total Mortality: A 25-Year Follow-Up Study of 255 Physicians," *Psychosomatic Medicine* 45, no. 1 (March 1983): 59–63, https://www.ncbi.nlm.nih.gov/pubmed/6844529.

Chapter 8. Sleep: A Vital Component of Health

1. University of Chicago Medical Center, "New Study Shows People Sleep Even Less Than They Think," *ScienceDaily*, July 3, 2006, www.sciencedaily.com/releases/2006/07/060703162945.htm.

2. P. Wang et al., "Night-Shift Work, Sleep Duration, Daytime Napping, and Breast Cancer Risk," *Sleep Medicine* 16, no. 4 (April 2015): 462–68, doi:10.1016/j.sleep.2014.11.017.

3. M. Rööst and P. Nilsson, "Sleep Disorders — A Public Health Problem: Potential Risk Factor in the Development of Type 2 Diabetes, Hypertension, Dyslipidemia, and Premature Aging," *Lakartidningen*

99, no. 3 (January 2002): 154–57, https://www.ncbi.nlm.nih.gov/pubmed/11838069.

4. F. P. Cappuccio et al., "Quantity and Quality of Sleep and Incidence of Type 2 Diabetes: A Systematic Review and Meta-analysis," *Diabetes Care* 33, no. 2 (February 2010): 414–20, doi:10.2337/dc09-1124.

5. S. Taheri et al., "Short Sleep Duration Is Associated with Reduced Leptin, Elevated Ghrelin, and Increased Body Mass Index," *PLoS Medicine* 1, no. 3 (December 2004): e62, doi:10.1371/journal.pmed.0010062.

6. A. A. Prather et al., "Behaviorally Assessed Sleep and Susceptibility to the Common Cold," *Sleep* 38, no. 9 (September 2015): 1353–59, doi: 10.5665/sleep.4968.

7. K. E. West et al., "Blue Light from Light-Emitting Diodes Elicits a Dose-Dependent Suppression of Melatonin in Humans," *Journal of Applied Physiology* 110, no. 3 (March 2011): 619–26, doi:10.1152/japplphysiol.01413.2009.

Chapter 9. Battling Environmental Enemies

1. Amy Roeder, "Harmful, Untested Chemicals Rife in Personal Care Products," Harvard School of Public Health, February 13, 2014, https://www.hsph.harvard.edu/news/features/harmful-chemicals-in-personal-care-products.

2. M. V. Maffini et al., "Endocrine Disruptors and Reproductive Health: The Case of Bisphenol-A," *Molecular and Cellular Endocrinology* 254–55 (July 25, 2006): 179–86, doi:10.1016/j.mce.2006.04.033; E. Makaji et al., "Effect of Environmental Contaminants on Beta Cell Function," *International Journal of Toxicology* 30, no. 4 (August 2011): 410–18, doi:10.1177/1091581811405544.

3. Julia R. Barrett, "Chemical Exposures: The Ugly Side of Beauty Products," *Environmental Health Perspectives* 113, no. 1 (January 2005): A24, https://www.ncbi.nlm.nih.gov/pmc/articles/PMC1253722.

4. J. Jurewicz et al., "Exposure to Widespread Environmental Endocrine Disrupting Chemicals and Human Sperm Sex Ratio," *Environmental Pollution* 213 (June 2016): 732–40, doi:10.1016/j.envpol.2016.02.008.

5. J. Boberg et al., "Possible Endocrine Disrupting Effects of Parabens and Their Metabolites," *Reproductive Toxicology* 30, no. 2 (September 2010): 301–12, doi:10.1016/j.reprotox.2010.03.011.

6. Shawn Pan et al., "Parabens and Human Epidermal Growth Factor

Receptor Ligands Cross-Talk in Breast Cancer Cells," *Environmental Health Perspectives* 124, no. 5 (May 2016), doi:10.1289/ehp.1409200.

7. D. Mukerjee, "Health Impact of Polychlorinated Dibenzo-P-Dioxins: A Critical Review," *Journal of the Air & Waste Management Association* 48, no. 2 (February 1998): 157–65, https://www.ncbi.nlm.nih.gov/pubmed/9517323.

8. Sally S. White and Linda S. Birnbaum, "An Overview of the Effects of Dioxins and Dioxin-Like Compounds on Vertebrates, as Documented in Human and Ecological Epidemiology," *Journal of Environmental Science and Health, Part C, Environmental Carcinogenesis and Ecotoxicology Reviews* 27, no. 4 (October 2009): 197–211, doi:10.1080/10590500903310047.

9. J. M. Kreitinger, C. A. Beamer, and D. M. Shepherd, "Environmental Immunology: Lessons Learned from Exposure to a Select Panel of Immunotoxicants," *Journal of Immunology* 196, no. 8 (April 2016): 3217–25, doi:10.4049/jimmunol.1502149.

10. T. B. Hayes et al., "Demasculinization and Feminization of Male Gonads by Atrazine: Consistent Effects across Vertebrate Classes," *Journal of Steroid Biochemistry and Molecular Biology* 127, nos. 1–2 (October 2011): 64–73, doi:10.1016/j.jsbmb.2011.03.015.

11. J. R. Roy, S. Chakraborty, and T. R. Chakraborty, "Estrogen-Like Endocrine Disrupting Chemicals Affecting Puberty in Humans: A Review," *Medical Science Monitor* 15, no. 6 (June 2009): RA137–45.

12. "Public Health Statement: Perfluoroalkyls," Agency for Toxic Substances and Disease Registry, Division of Toxicology and Human Health Sciences, August 2015, https://www.atsdr.cdc.gov/toxprofiles/tp200-c1-b.pdf.

13. G. Du et al., "Perfluorooctane Sulfonate (PFOS) Affects Hormone Receptor Activity, Steroidogenesis, and Expression of Endocrine-Related Genes In Vitro and In Vivo," *Environmental Toxicology and Chemistry* 32, no. 2 (February 2013): 353–60, https://www.ncbi.nlm.nih.gov/pubmed/23074026.

14. M. de Cock et al., "Prenatal Exposure to Endocrine Disrupting Chemical in Relation to Thyroid Hormone Levels in Infants: A Dutch Prospective Cohort Study," *Environmental Health* 13 (December 10, 2014): 106, doi:10.1186/1476-069X-13-106.

15. A. A. López-Cepero and C. Palacios, "Association of the Intestinal Microbiota and Obesity." *Puerto Rico Health Sciences Journal* 34,

no. 2 (June 2015): 60–64, https://www.ncbi.nlm.nih.gov/pubmed/26061054.

16. A. H. Smith et al., "Cancer Risks from Arsenic in Drinking Water," *Environmental Health Perspectives* 97 (July 1992): 259–67.

17. "EWG's 2017 Shopper's Guide to Pesticides in Produce," Environmental Working Group, https://www.ewg.org/foodnews/summary.php.

18. Ibid.

Chapter 10. Superfoods and Supplements

1. S. E. Power et al., "Intestinal Microbiota, Diet, and Health," *British Journal of Nutrition* 111, no. 3 (February 2014): 387–402, doi:10.1017/S0007114513002560.

2. I. T. Johnson, "Glucosinolates: Bioavailability and Importance to Health," *International Journal for Vitamin and Nutrition Research* 72, no. 1 (January 2002): 26–31, doi:10.1024/0300-9831.72.1.26.

3. H. Tilg and A. R. Moschen, "Microbiota and Diabetes: An Evolving Relationship," *Gut* 63, no. 9 (September 2014): 1513–21, doi:10.1136/gutjnl-2014-306928.

4. S. Sivaprakasam, P. D. Prasad, and N. Singh, "Benefits of Short-Chain Fatty Acids and Their Receptors in Inflammation and Carcinogenesis," *Pharmacology & Therapeutics* 164 (August 2016): 144–51, doi: 10.1016/j.pharmthera.2016.04.007.

5. Cristina Lull, Harry J. Wichers, and Huub F. J. Savelkoul, "Anti-inflammatory and Immunomodulating Properties of Fungal Metabolites," *Mediators of Inflammation* 2005, no. 2 (June 9, 2005): 63–80, doi:10.1155/MI.2005.63.

6. C. M. Albert et al., "Nut Consumption and Decreased Risk of Sudden Cardiac Death in the Physicians' Health Study," *Archives of Internal Medicine* 162, no. 12 (June 24, 2002): 1382–87, https://www.ncbi.nlm.nih.gov/pubmed/12076237.

7. N. Maithili Karpaga Selvi et al., "Efficacy of Turmeric as Adjuvant Therapy in Type 2 Diabetic Patients," *Indian Journal of Clinical Biochemistry* 30, no. 2 (April 2015): 180–86, doi:10.1007/s12291-014-0436-2; G. Ramadan and O. El-Menshawy, "Protective Effects of Ginger-Turmeric Rhizomes Mixture on Joint Inflammation, Atherogenesis, Kidney Dysfunction, and Other Complications in a Rat

Model of Human Rheumatoid Arthritis," *International Journal of Rheumatic Diseases* 16, no. 2 (April 2013): 219–29, doi:10.1111/1756-185X.12054; and B. B. Aggarwal, S. C. Gupta, and B. Sung, "Curcumin: An Orally Bioavailable Blocker of TNF and Other Pro-inflammatory Biomarkers," *British Journal of Pharmacology* 169, no. 8 (August 2013): 1672–92, doi:10.1111/bph.12131.

8. Solomon Habtemariam, "The Therapeutic Potential of Rosemary (*Rosmarinus officinalis*) Diterpenes for Alzheimer's Disease," *Evidence-Based Complementary and Alternative Medicine* 2016 (2016), doi:10.1155/2016/2680409.

9. K. Puangsombat, W. Jirapakkul, and J. S. Smith, "Inhibitory Activity of Asian Spices on Heterocyclic Amines Formation in Cooked Beef Patties," *Journal of Food Science* 76, no. 8 (October 2011): T174–80, doi:10.1111/j.1750-3841.2011.02338.x.

10. R. Grzanna, L. Lindmark, and C. G. Frondoza, "Ginger: An Herbal Medicinal Product with Broad Anti-inflammatory Actions," *Journal of Medicinal Food* 8, no. 2 (Summer 2005): 125–32.

11. S. P. Dibazar, S. Fateh, and S. Daneshmandi, "Immunomodulatory Effects of Clove (*Syzygium aromaticum*) Constituents on Macrophages: In Vitro Evaluations of Aqueous and Ethanolic Components," *Journal of Immunotoxicology* 12, no. 2 (April–June 2015): 124–31, doi:10.3109/1547691X.2014.912698.

12. S. K. Ghawi, L. Methven, and K. Niranjan, "The Potential to Intensify Sulforaphane Formation in Cooked Broccoli (*Brassica oleracea var. italica*) Using Mustard Seeds (*Sinapis alba*)," *Food Chemistry* 138, nos. 2–3 (June 1, 2013): 1734–41, doi:10.1016/j.foodchem.2012.10.119.

13. C. A. Martins et al., "Curcumin in Combination with Piperine Suppresses Osteoclastogenesis In Vitro," *Journal of Endodontics* 41, no. 10 (October 2015): 1638–45, doi:10.1016/j.joen.2015.05.009.

14. R. W. Allen et al., "Cinnamon Use in Type 2 Diabetes: An Updated Systematic Review and Meta-analysis," *Annals of Family Medicine* 11, no. 5 (September–October 2013): 452–59, doi:10.1370/afm.1517.

15. K. Y. Forrest and W. L. Stuhldreher, "Prevalence and Correlates of Vitamin D Deficiency in US Adults," *Nutrition Research* 31, no. 1 (January 2011): 48–54, doi:10.1016/j.nutres.2010.12.001.

16. M. Ashkanian, E. Tehrani, and P. Videbech, "The Effect of Vitamin D on Neuropsychiatric Conditions," *Ugeskrift for Laeger* 172, no. 17

(April 26, 2010): 1296–300, https://www.ncbi.nlm.nih.gov/pub med/20444398.

17. J. Welsh, "Vitamin D and Cancer: Integration of Cellular Biology, Molecular Mechanisms, and Animal Models," *Scandinavian Journal of Clinical and Laboratory Investigation, Supplementum* 243 (2012): 103–11, doi:10.3109/00365513.2012.682870.

18. Simon C. Dyall, "Long-Chain Omega-3 Fatty Acids and the Brain: A Review of the Independent and Shared Effects of EPA, DPA, and DHA," *Frontiers in Aging Neuroscience* 7 (April 21, 2015): 52, doi: 10.3389/fnagi.2015.00052.

19. A. J. Sinclair, K. J. Murphy, and D. Li, "Marine Lipids: Overview 'News Insights and Lipid Composition of Lyprinol,'" *Allergie et Immunologie* 32, no. 7 (September 2000): 261–71, https://www.ncbi .nlm.nih.gov/pubmed/11094639.

20. Tommy Cederholm, Norman Salem Jr., and Jan Palmblad, "Omega-3 Fatty Acids in the Prevention of Cognitive Decline in Humans," *Advances in Nutrition* 4, no. 6 (November 6, 2013): 672–76, doi:10.3945/an.113.004556.

21. A. Rosanoff, C. M. Weaver, and R. K. Rude, "Suboptimal Magnesium Status in the United States: Are the Health Consequences Underestimated?" *Nutrition Reviews* 70, no. 3 (March 2012): 153–64, doi:10.1111/j.1753-4887.2011.00465.x.

22. M. Banach et al., "Statin Therapy and Plasma Coenzyme Q10 Concentrations: A Systematic Review and Meta-analysis of Placebo-Controlled Trials," *Pharmacological Research* 99 (September 2015): 329–36, doi:10.1016/j.phrs.2015.07.008.

23. N. Suksomboon, N. Poolsup, and A. Yuwanakorn, "Systematic Review and Meta-analysis of the Efficacy and Safety of Chromium Supplementation in Diabetes," *Journal of Clinical Pharmacy and Therapeutics* 39, no. 3 (June 2014): 292–306, doi:10.1111/jcpt.12147.

24. C. S. Johnston, C. M. Kim, and A. J. Buller, "Vinegar Improves Insulin Sensitivity to a High-Carbohydrate Meal in Subjects with Insulin Resistance or Type 2 Diabetes," *Diabetes Care* 27, no. 1 (January 2004): 281–82, https://www.ncbi.nlm.nih.gov/pubmed/14694010.

Index

Page references containing an italicized *fig.* indicate illustrations or material contained in their captions. Page references containing an italicized *t.* indicate tables.

abdominal obesity, 18–19, 19 *t. 1.1.*
  See also belly fat
abs, six-pack, 112, 119
acceptance, 139–40
acesulfame, 53
acid reflux, 182
activity thermogenesis (AT), 102, 103 *fig. 6.1*
advertising, 78
alcohol: avoidance of, 4, 52, 54–55, 92, 159; dehydrating effect of, 98; facts/fallacies, 57; health risks of, 54–55, 57, 237; sleep deprivation and, 159
algae, 184
allergens, 69–70
almond butter: Breakfast Bowl, Turbo Metabolism, 190; Dressing, Ginger Almond, 199; "Risotto," Lemon Cauliflower, 232; Smoothie, Scrumptious, 194
almond milk: Cauliflower Fettucine "Alfredo," 225–26; Dressing, Ginger Almond, 199; Eggplant Mole with Quinoa, 219–20; Oatmeal to Go, No-Cook Strawberry, 192; Pasta, Roasted Romanesco Cauliflower and Asparagus, 227–28; Soup, Thai Hot-and-Sour, 201–2; Sweet Potatoes, Mashed, and Spinach, 216
almonds: Dressing, Ginger Almond, 199; "Risotto," Lemon Cauliflower, 232; Salad, Simply Delicious, 198; as snack option, 195
Aloo Beans, 203
Aloo Gobhi, 204–5
alpha lipoic acid, 185, 186
Alzheimer's disease, 17, 23–24, 62, 71, 170, 182
amygdala, 142
animal fats, 172

About the Author

Pankaj Vij, MD, is passionate about nutrition, fitness, and human performance. He is on a quest to help people slow down the aging process and optimize human performance, thereby enhancing *health span*, not just life span. He practices what he preaches by eating a low-glycemic, anti-inflammatory, real-food diet; getting regular physical activity; meditating; and sleeping well. He adds music and humor for good measure.

Board certified in internal medicine and obesity medicine, Dr. Vij has been practicing medicine since 1997. He has helped thousands of people achieve and maintain their goal weight and improve their fitness level, thus helping them live healthier and longer with fewer medications.

When he is not working, he spends time outdoors with his family and plays guitar and African drums. Dr. Vij is an active volunteer, helping the medically underserved in Central and South America and Asia.

You can learn more and reach Dr. Vij through his personal health websites, DoctorVij.com and HealthZoneLife.com. HealthZone Life (cosponsored with Dr. Douglas Amis) teaches that health is the new wealth. The objective of this project is to position you to win the best life for yourself and your family.

NEW WORLD LIBRARY is dedicated to publishing books and other media that inspire and challenge us to improve the quality of our lives and the world.

We are a socially and environmentally aware company. We recognize that we have an ethical responsibility to our customers, our staff members, and our planet.

We serve our customers by creating the finest publications possible on personal growth, creativity, spirituality, wellness, and other areas of emerging importance. We serve New World Library employees with generous benefits, significant profit sharing, and constant encouragement to pursue their most expansive dreams.

As a member of the Green Press Initiative, we print an increasing number of books with soy-based ink on 100 percent postconsumer-waste recycled paper. Also, we power our offices with solar energy and contribute to non-profit organizations working to make the world a better place for us all.

Our products are available in bookstores everywhere.

www.newworldlibrary.com

At NewWorldLibrary.com you can download our catalog,
subscribe to our e-newsletter, read our blog,
and link to authors' websites, videos, and podcasts.

Find us on Facebook, follow us on Twitter, and watch us on YouTube.

Send your questions and comments our way!
You make it possible for us to do what we love to do.

Phone: 415-884-2100 or 800-972-6657
Catalog requests: Ext. 10 | Orders: Ext. 10 | Fax: 415-884-2199
escort@newworldlibrary.com

NEW WORLD LIBRARY
publishing books that change lives   14 Pamaron Way, Novato, CA 94949